The Clinical Anaesthesia Viva Book

The Clinical Anaesthesia Viva Book

by

Simon J. Mills MB ChB MRCP FRCA
Specialist Registrar in Anaesthesia
North West Rotation

Simon L. Maguire MB ChB FRCA
Specialist Registrar in Anaesthesia
North West Rotation

Julian M. Barker MB ChB MRCP FRCA
Specialist Registrar in Anaesthesia
North West Rotation

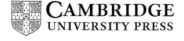
CAMBRIDGE
UNIVERSITY PRESS

CAMBRIDGE UNIVERSITY PRESS
Cambridge, New York, Melbourne, Madrid, Cape Town, Singapore, São Paulo

Cambridge University Press
The Edinburgh Building, Cambridge CB2 8RU, UK

Published in the United States of America by Cambridge University Press, New York

www.cambridge.org
Information on this title: www.cambridge.org/9780521676953

First published 2002
Reprinted 2003, 2005
Reprinted by Cambridge University Press 2005
Third printing 2007

Printed in the United Kingdom at the University Press, Cambridge

A catalogue record for this publication is available from the British Library

ISBN-13 978-0-521-67695-3 paperback

Contents

Introduction

There are many books available on the market dealing with the final FRCA examination. The vast majority of these cover multiple choice, short answer questions and the clinical science vivas. During our revision we were disappointed by the lack of books aimed specifically at the clinical vivas.

We have produced a book of long and short clinical viva questions based on previous candidates' recollections from the final examination. Having surveyed Specialist Registrars in the North West region who have recently taken the final FRCA, we hope the questions are an accurate representation of questions that have appeared in the examination. The answers have been constructed from a combination of popular textbooks, recent publications (typically review articles and editorials) and the experiences of the candidates (depending on how they fared!).

The results of the survey demonstrated that many scenarios have appeared frequently over the past couple of years, for example 'awareness'. However, the line of questioning has varied from one set of examiners to the next. Our answers have been constructed to try to cover these different avenues of questioning. This explains why some of the short viva answers contain considerably more information than could possibly be delivered in a 5-minute viva.

The 15 long cases have been selected to cover common recurring themes such as the difficult airway, preoptimisation and the regional versus GA debate.

The book also contains hints and techniques for revision and conduct during the examination.

Mills S
Maguire S
Barker J
November 2001

Foreword

One of the first aims of every trainee on entering the specialist registrar grade is to pass the Final FRCA examination at the earliest opportunity. The decision to take it as soon as possible must be balanced with the realisation that preparation must be adequate and that takes time. It is not an easy examination as it tests a considerable breadth and depth of knowledge – as it should.

Every candidate has, of course, to have an adequate basic factual knowledge. This is gained from many sources, in particular books, courses and experience. All parts of the examination test factual knowledge. The vivas, however, also test how those facts can be assembled to solve problems and to discuss the merits and demerits of these potential solutions. It is widely believed that there is a 'knack' to passing the vivas and that you might know enough but if you don't have the 'knack', you might be unlucky.

There are many ways to study but one which seems to work well for many candidates is the group learning process. This self-directed, problem-based learning approach is finding its way into the undergraduate curriculum of many medical schools. The group need only be two people but the process of asking each other questions and trying to give a coherent answer is a useful learning process for both. The problem which besets candidates is how do you know that what you are asking each other is realistic and is pitched at the correct level? That is where this book comes in.

The authors of this book are specialist registrars who have sat and passed the Final FRCA examination relatively recently and therefore have a feel for the sort of questions which were asked. These memories, together with those of some colleagues, have been rebuilt into questions which are realistic and can be used as a basis for revision. Example answers are included, but it must be remembered that there are many possible answers to each scenario and the ones given here may not be all that an examiner would want. Also, lest any future candidate obtain the wrong impression, the questions are realistic but they are not actually verbatim from the real bank. Remember that this book should not be used as simply a reading book but as a basis for discussion, thought and practice.

The bottom line is that this book will prove to be of use to any candidate sitting the Final FRCA examination clinical vivas. It will not, however, tell you all of the questions with all possible combinations of the correct answers. And you still need to know what you are talking about! Good Luck!

Brian J Pollard, Professor of Anaesthesia,
Manchester Royal Infirmary,
Oxford Road, Manchester, M13 9WL

Acknowledgements

The authors would like to express their sincere thanks for the contributors made to the book by the following:

For advice and encouragement:

- Professor B Pollard, Professor of Anaesthesia, University Department of Anaesthesia, Manchester Royal Infirmary

For taking the time to answer questions about their viva experiences:

- The specialist Registrars in Anaesthesia, North Western rotation

For their assistance with the chest X-rays:

- Dr A Khan, Consultant Radiologist, North Manchester General Hospital
- Dr C Jones, Consultant Radiologist, North Manchester General Hospital
- Dr R Bissett, Consultant Radiologist, North Manchester General Hospital
- Dr R Sawyer, Consultant Radiologist, Wythenshawe Hospital
- Dr C Barker, Specialist Registrar in Radiology, Manchester
- Dr I Macartney, Consultant Anaesthetist, North Manchester General Hospital
- Dr C Coutinho, Consultant Radiologist, Royal Preston Hospital

For their assistance with the ECGs and pulmonary function tests:

- The staff of the Cardiorespiratory department, North Manchester General Hospital
- Mr K Pearce, Chief Clinical Scientific Officer, Cardiology department, Wythenshawe Hospital

For assistance with the chronic pain questions:

- Dr K Grady, Consultant Anaesthetist, Wythenshawe Hospital

We would also like to thank the publishers, Greenwich Medical Media Ltd.

Chapter 1

Preparation for the Clinical Viva

Examination format

You need to be aware of the format of the vivas.
The day consists of two viva sessions:

The clinical viva

This lasts 50 minutes and consists of a long case and three short cases or scenarios. During the first ten minutes you will have the opportunity to view clinical information related to the long case consisting of history, examination findings and investigations e.g. ECG, chest X-ray, pulmonary function tests and blood results. This is followed by 20 minutes of questioning related to this case. During the final 20 minutes the examiners will question you on three further unrelated topics.

The clinical science viva

This is a 30 minute viva consisting of questions on applied pharmacology, anatomy, physiology and physics. This viva is not within the scope of this book.

An approach to revision for the clinical viva

The period between the written paper and viva examination is a stressful time. For the first two weeks you do not even know if you have a viva. This makes it difficult to find the motivation to carry on working until the results are posted. The last thing you want to do is continue the cold, factual learning that has made your life such a misery over the last few weeks. You want to go to the pub instead! However, if you are 'invited' to attend for the vivas, you will find yourself wishing you had worked solidly for the two weeks since the written paper! What is needed is a change of tack in order to sustain the flagging momentum. We found sitting around in armchairs (cups of tea in hand) discussing anaesthetic topics far preferable to the 'textbook and solitary desk-lamp at midnight' scenario.

It is important to realise that the viva requires a different approach to revision. This book aims to give you a strategy for viva revision that will hopefully make it less tedious.

We initially found our viva technique left much to be desired, despite adequate knowledge. There is a particular 'knack' to passing this type of examination and possessing a well-honed technique can enable you to appear confident and knowledgeable (even if you don't feel it!). With the experience you have gained as a trainee, your knowledge base is very likely to be good enough to tackle most questions. However, it is the way in which you *communicate* your knowledge that will need to impress the examiners. As in all branches of anaesthesia there are many ways to skin a cat, and revising for the clinical viva is no exception. We found the following techniques extremely valuable in the run-up to the vivas:

- **Group revision**
- **Frequent practice**
- **Practise categorising**
- **Card system**

Group revision

It is extremely useful to team up with some friends or colleagues regularly in the weeks before the viva and practise talking about anaesthetic topics. Practising with friends has several advantages:

- The whole exam period is very stressful and seeing your friends on a regular basis will help keep you sane. This is better than locking yourself in a small room with a pile of books and trying to learn the coagulation cascade for the fifth time since qualification!
- Your morale will remain in better shape than if you were revising on your own because you will be able to encourage each other. You will also be more aware of the progress you are making.
- As a group you can pool your resources in terms of reference books and previous questions. During the working day one of you may have had a practice viva with a consultant who asked an awkward question or a common question asked in a different way. You can then discuss with your friends how they would have answered it.
- Different people revise in different ways and consequently will have their own way of talking about a subject. This means that others in the group will benefit from listening to the practice viva. They may have a particular piece of knowledge that really helps an answer gel together or they may use a particular turn-of-phrase that succinctly deals with a potential minefield.
- You can practise phrasing your answers in a particular way in the knowledge that if it all falls apart halfway through, it won't matter and you can have another go. This is less easy to do in front of consultants who might write your reference!
- By being 'the examiner' you will gain insight into the pitfalls of the viva process. You can usually see someone digging a hole for themselves a mile off!

Frequent practice

Repetition of clinical scenarios

During your revision you will find the same clinical situations coming up time and time again (as in the exam). Over the years anaesthetic techniques may change but new techniques are all aimed at trying to solve particular *clinical problems*, for example the fibreoptic scope to help with the difficult airway or new drugs that provide more cardiovascular stability. However, the *problems* remain the same! Patients will still present with difficult airways, ischaemic heart disease, COAD, obesity, hypertension etc. The more you practise, the more often you will find yourself repeating the problems each of these scenarios presents and thus the more confident and slick you will become at delivering the salient points.

There are obviously a few exceptions, e.g. MRI scanners and laser surgery, where the advancement of technology has presented new challenges to the anaesthetist. These situations are in the minority and as long as you are aware of them and the associated anaesthetic problems, you should be well equipped to deal with questions on them in the exam.

The clinical scenarios break down into a few categories:

- **Medical** conditions that have anaesthetic implications e.g.
    Aortic stenosis
    Diabetes
    Hyperthyroidism
- **Surgical** procedures that have anaesthetic implications e.g.
    Oesophagectomy
    CABG
    Pneumonectomy
- **Anaesthetic** emergencies/difficult situations e.g.
    Anaphylaxis
    Malignant hyperthermia
    Failed intubation
- **Paediatric** cases. These represent a limited range of cases the examiners are likely to ask you about e.g.
    Upper airway obstruction
    Pyloric stenosis
    Bleeding tonsil

Having repeatedly practised these clinical scenarios you will soon realise that the problems of anaesthetising an obese patient with diabetes, ischaemic heart disease, porphyria and myasthenia for an abdominal aortic aneurysm repair(!) can be broken down into the problems that the respective conditions present to the anaesthetist plus the problems of the specific operation. You may then approach what seems to be a nightmare question with a degree of confidence and structure.

Phrasing

It cannot be over-emphasised that frequent practice will improve your viva technique. As already mentioned, some topics crop up again and again in different situations, such as part of a long case or even a complete short case (e.g. obesity, anaesthesia for the elderly or the difficult airway). With regular practice you will soon develop your own 'patter' to help you deal with these common clinical scenarios. These can then be adopted at opportune moments to buy yourself easy marks whilst actually giving you time to gather your thoughts.

Practise categorising

Putting order to your answers demonstrates to the examiners that you conduct your clinical practice in a systematic and safe way. If you do not mention the most important points first (e.g. airway problems in a patient presenting with a goitre) then this may suggest to the examiners that you are disorganised. An 'ABC' (order of priority) approach to many of the questions may be helpful. For example, in obese patients managing the airway has a higher priority than difficulty with cannulation.

It is often a good idea to use your opening sentence to tell the examiners how you are going to categorise your answer.

Example 1:

'*Tell me about the anaesthetic implications of rheumatoid arthritis.*'

'Patients with rheumatoid arthritis may have a difficult airway and secondary respiratory and cardiovascular pathology. They are frequently anaemic, taking immunosuppressant drugs, and the severe joint pathology leads to problems with positioning.'

Example 2:

'*What are the important considerations when anaesthetising a patient for a pneumonectomy?*'

'These may be divided into three broad areas: the *preoperative* assessment of fitness for pneumonectomy and optimisation, the *conduct of anaesthesia* with particular reference to one-lung anaesthesia, positioning, intraoperative monitoring and fluid balance and finally *postoperative care.*'

Card system

We formatted postcards to summarise the main problems associated with different anaesthetic situations. These proved to be a good starting point for viva practice and a quick source of reference. They also encouraged us to deliver the first few points in a punchy manner.

For example:

'*What problems do you anticipate when anaesthetising a patient with Down's syndrome?*'

'These patients present the following problems for the anaesthetist. They may have a difficult airway, an unstable neck, cardiac abnormalities, mental retardation, epilepsy and a high incidence of hepatitis B infection.'

Viva technique

- **Think first**
- **The opening sentence**
- **Categorise or die!**
- **The long case**

Think first

Don't panic. If you are unlucky enough to be asked a question about an obscure subject such as lithium therapy (as two of us were in our science viva) remember the examiners have only just seen the questions as well. It may also be of some comfort to know that there will be at least ten other candidates being asked the same question at the same time. Keep things simple at first and think about how you are going to structure your answer. Categorising your answer may allow you to deliver more information about the topic than you thought you knew. Conversely, do not dwell on what you do not know e.g. the pH and dose!

Example: *'Tell me about lithium'*

Think . . .	'What is it used for?'
Say . . .	'Lithium is a drug used in the treatment of mania and the prophylaxis of manic depression.'

Think . . .	'What is the presentation and dose? . . . I don't know the dose.'
Say . . .	'It is presented in tablet-form.'

Think . . .	'What is its mode of action? . . . I have no idea but I know it is an antipsychotic!'
Say . . .	'Its main action is as an antipsychotic.'

Think . . .	'Why are they asking me this question? What is the relevance to anaesthetic practice?'
Say . . .	'It has a narrow therapeutic range and therefore toxicity must be looked for. Side-effects may include nausea, vomiting, convulsions, arrhythmias and diabetes insipidus with hypernatraemia.'

A similar approach can be used for the clinical viva.

The opening sentence

This will set the tone of the viva. If the first words to come from your mouth are poorly structured, ill thought-out or just plain rubbish then you are likely to annoy the examiners and will face an uphill struggle. If, on the other hand, your first sentence is coherent, succinct and structured then you will be half way there. With a bit of luck the examiners will sit back, breathe a sigh of relief (because it has been a very long day for them) and allow you to demonstrate your obvious knowledge of the subject in hand!

For example:

> *'What are the problems associated with anaesthesia for thyroid disease?'*

> 'Anaesthesia for patients with thyroid disease has implications in the pre-, intra- and postoperative periods.'

You are then able to expand in a logical way from here.

> 'Preoperatively, assessment of the airway and control of the functional activity of the gland is essential...'

Categorise or die!

Remember this lends structure to your answer and gives the examiners the impression you are about to talk about the subject with authority. If you categorise your answer well enough they may actually stop you and move onto something else.

The long case

The above points relate to the short and long cases but there are aspects of the long case that can be anticipated. Some answers can therefore be prepared in advance.

Opening question

You will be asked to summarise the case so prepare your opening sentence beforehand.

For example:

> You may be asked to summarise the scenario of a 75-year-old man with chronic obstructive pulmonary disease who is scheduled to undergo an elective cardio-oesophagectomy the following day.

> *'Would you like to summarise the case?'*

> One possible answer may begin:

> 'This is an elderly gentleman with complex medical problems who is scheduled for a cardio-oesophagectomy. He has evidence of chronic obstructive pulmonary disease, ischaemic heart disease and diabetes. There will be substantial strain on his cardio-respiratory system. This operation is a major procedure that involves considerable fluid shifts, a potential for large blood loss and requires careful attention to analgesia. These are the main issues that I would concentrate on in my preoperative assessment.'

Even though a cardio-oesophagectomy involves other considerations (e.g. double-lumen tube/one-lung ventilation) it can be seen that this opening sentence could be adapted to suit other clinical scenarios such as:

- Pneumonectomy
- Laparotomy
- CABG/Valve replacement
- Cystectomy
- Open prostatectomy

Analyse *all* the investigations

You will be asked for your opinion on the ECG, chest X-ray, blood results etc. so make sure you have decided on the abnormalities and the most likely causes for them in the 10 minutes you have to view the data. Try to make your answers punchy and authoritative.

For example:

> 'The ECG shows sinus rhythm with a rate of 80 and an old inferior infarct' is better than going through the ECG in a painstaking 'The rate is ... the rhythm is ... the axis is ...'.

Don't waste valuable time waffling on about the normal-looking bones on a chest X-ray if there is a barn-door left lower lobe collapse. This does not necessarily imply you are not thorough providing you demonstrate that you have looked for and excluded other abnormalities.

Anaesthetic technique

You will usually be asked how you would anaesthetise the patient in the long case. There will often not be a right or wrong answer but you should try to decide on *your* technique and be able to justify it. The examiners may only be looking for the principles of anaesthesia for a particular condition such as aortic stenosis although this is probably more likely in the short cases.

For example:

> *'You are asked to provide an anaesthetic for a 77-year-old lady who needs a hemi-arthroplasty for a fractured neck of femur. She had a myocardial infarction 3 months ago and has evidence of heart failure.'*

You should be able to summarise the principles involved and choose an anaesthetic technique appropriate to the problems presented. You could, for example, give this patient a general anaesthetic with invasive monitoring (PAFC, A-line, etc.), you could use TIVA with remifentanil or a neuroaxial block. All of these techniques could be justified but to simply say that you would use propofol, fentanyl and a laryngeal mask without saying why may be asking for trouble!

In some circumstances it may be the options for management rather than a *specific* technique that is required. You may find it appropriate to list the options for analgesia in a patient having a pneumonectomy, for example, and then say why you would use one technique over the others.

You should try to address the anaesthetic technique for the long case **before** you face the examiners. You will not look very credible if you have had 10 minutes to decide on this and have not reached some kind of conclusion.

Overall, most candidates felt that the examiners were pleasant and generally helpful. If you are getting sidetracked they will probably give you a hint so you do not waste time talking about something for which there are no allocated marks. If they do give you a hint, take it!

Good luck.

Chapter 2

The Short Cases

Abdominal aortic aneurysm rupture ✓

You are called to the ward to see a 74-year-old man with a ruptured aortic aneurysm. His blood pressure is 70/40.

What are the major problems in managing a ruptured AAA?

Pre-operatively
- Severe hypovolaemia
- Initial fluid resuscitation must be cautious
- Assessment of concomitant medical problems
- No time for lengthy investigations
- Access to vascular surgery – may need to transfer out

Intra-operatively
- Cardiovascular instability
  - Induction
  - Before aortic cross-clamping
  - When the clamp is removed
- Large blood losses — Blood, FFP and platelets required
- Effects of massive transfusion
- Temperature control
- Metabolic acidosis

Post-operatively
- **Respiratory support** may be required for poor gas exchange and metabolic acidosis
- **Cardiovascular complications** include haemorrhage, myocardial and lower limb ischaemia
- **Renal failure** is common due to peri-operative hypotension, aortic cross-clamping (infra-renal clamp still significantly reduces renal blood-flow), atheromatous emboli, surgical insult, or intra-abdominal hypertension (>15 mmHg) or compartment syndrome (>25 mmHg)
- **Neurological sequelae** such as paraplegia or stroke may occur secondary to damaged spinal arteries or embolic/ischaemic events

What is your immediate management on the ward?

- ABC approach – highest FiO$_2$ obtainable should be commenced
- Two large-bore intravenous cannulae should be inserted and fluids given

How much fluid would you use?

This would depend on the blood pressure and the clinical state of the patient. A patient who has an unrecordable blood pressure and is about to arrest should be given fluids quickly but in this man **fluids should be given cautiously**. One should not necessarily aim to restore blood pressure to 'normal' as this may perpetuate the bleeding.

What else would you do?

- Take blood for full blood count, urea and electrolytes, clotting screen
- Cross-match for 10 units
- Second anaesthetist (preferably consultant) is required
- Haematology should be alerted to the need for large volumes of blood, FFP and platelets
- An assessment of co-existing medical problems and the likelihood of difficult intubation should be made
- **Do not delay surgery** whilst awaiting lengthy investigations
  Transfer the patient to the operating theatre as soon as possible

What monitoring would you use?

- ECG, non-invasive BP, SpO$_2$ and capnography initially
- **Surgery should not be delayed by prolonged attempts to insert arterial and central lines at this stage**

How would you proceed with anaesthesia?

- **Big drips**
- All vaso-active drugs should be drawn up prior to induction
- Blood should be immediately available
- A method of delivering warmed fluids rapidly and continuously is beneficial such as a 'Level-1™ infusor'
- **Anaesthetise in theatre on the table**
- A rapid sequence induction is performed with the **surgeon scrubbed** and the **patient already cleaned and draped**
- Anaesthesia is maintained with an appropriate agent in oxygen/air
- Avoid nitrous oxide because bowel distension may increase intra-abdominal pressure post-operatively
- When the cross-clamp is on and there is 'relative' stability, invasive lines may be inserted if not already in place
- Temperature probe
- Nasogastric tube

■ Active warming such as with a warm air blower over the chest helps to maintain temperature but should be avoided on the legs during clamping

■ **Renoprotective therapy** – renal impairment is common following aortic surgery. The infusion of mannitol (0.5 g/kg) or dopamine prior to cross-clamping may help to preserve renal function. Recently, infusion of **dopexamine** has also been shown to have a protective effect (at least in elective aortic surgery) and is less likely to produce the tachycardia associated with dopamine (due to less β_1 activity). It also has a protective effect on the splanchnic circulation

How would you control the hypertension associated with cross-clamping?

SVR may rise by up to 40% resulting in myocardial ischaemia. If increasing the inspired **volatile** concentration and giving **opioid** and/or **propofol** are not effective then **GTN** can be used, especially if myocardial ischaemia is present.

How would you manage the patient at the end of the operation?

■ **Intensive care** is usually required

■ Sedation and ventilation may need to be continued until the temperature is corrected, cardiovascular stability is established and acid–base status and gas exchange are acceptable

References
Morgan GE, Mikhail MS. *Clinical Anaesthesiology,* 2nd edition, 1996. Appleton and Lange, Stamford, CT

Nimmo AF. Anaesthesia for emergency abdominal aortic aneurysm surgery. *RCA Bulletin* 5, January 2001

Welch M, Newstead C, Smyth V, Dodd D, Walker G. Evaluation of dopexamine hydrochloride as a renoprotective agent during aortic surgery. *Annals of Vascular Surgery* 1995, Volume 9(5), p488–492

Acromegaly ✓

An acromegalic patient presents for surgery to a pituitary tumour.

What are the common surgical approaches?

There are two main approaches to surgery:

(1) Over 90% of pituitary adenomas will be treated by the **trans-sphenoidal approach**. This approach, in which an incision is made in the nasal septum, is well tolerated and gives good cosmetic results. Complications are uncommon but include:

■ Haemorrhage
■ Visual loss

■ Persistent CSF leak
■ Panhypopituitarism
■ Stroke

(2) The other surgical option is a **frontal craniotomy**.

How can pituitary tumours present?

Most pituitary tumours are benign and arise from the anterior pituitary. They can be secreting (around 75%) or non-secreting and may present in a number of ways:

■ Mass effect of the tumour: Headache
                                   Nausea and vomiting
                                   Visual field defects
                                   Cranial nerve palsies
                                   Papilloedema
                                   Raised ICP (rare, but more common with non-functioning macroadenomas)
■ Effects from the secretion of one or more hormones
■ Non-specific – headache, infertility, epilepsy
■ Incidental e.g. during imaging ('incidentalomas')

Classification of pituitary tumours:

1. **Non-functioning** (25%)	Commonly null-cell adenomas, craniopharyngiomas and meningiomas
2. **Functioning** (75%)	Prolactin 30%
	Prolactin + GH 10–12%
	GH 20%
	ACTH 12–15%
	FSH/LH 1–2%
	TSH 1%

What are the features of acromegaly?

There is hypersecretion of growth hormone with resultant soft tissue overgrowth. Clinical features include:

■ **Face**   Increased skull size
                                   Prominent supraorbital ridge
                                   Prognathism
                                   Headaches
■ **Mouth**   Macroglossia
                                   Soft tissue overgrowth in larynx/pharynx
                                   Obstructive sleep apnoea
■ **Skeleton**   Large hands and feet
                                   Thick skin
                                   Osteoporosis
                                   Kyphosis

- **Neuromuscular** RLN palsy
  Peripheral neuropathy
  Proximal myopathy
- **Cardiovascular** Hypertension
  Heart failure
- **Endocrine** Diabetes

> **Diagnostic tests for acromegaly:**
>
> - Random serum growth hormone >10 mU/L – can give false positives due to its short half-life and pattern of release
> - Failure of growth hormone suppression following a glucose load
> - Elevated IGF-1 – growth hormone exerts many of its effects through insulin-like growth factor-1 (IGF-1) which also has a longer half-life than growth hormone

Which features are of concern to the anaesthetist?

- **Upper airway obstruction** This may result from a large mandible, tongue and epiglottis together with generalised mucosal hypertrophy. Laryngeal narrowing may cause difficulty with tracheal intubation, and postoperative respiratory obstruction can occur. A history of stridor, hoarseness, dyspnoea or obstructive sleep apnoea should be specifically asked for
- **Cardiac** Hypertension and congestive cardiac failure requiring preoperative investigation and treatment
- **Endocrine** Commonly glucose intolerance and diabetes mellitus. Other associations include thyroid and adrenal abnormalities that may necessitate thyroxine and steroid replacement

What postoperative management problems may you encounter?

- **Surgical** complications such as: Haemorrhage
  Stroke
  Visual loss

- **Hormonal supplementation**
  Steroids Surgery may reduce the function of the pituitary gland and hydrocortisone is often prescribed in the immediate perioperative phase
  Thyroxine Prescribed with caution due to the risk of cardiac ischaemia
  Insulin Titrated to the required serum glucose concentration

■ **Diabetes insipidus**
This occurs in 40% of patients and is transient, typically occurring in the first 12–24 hours due to oedema around the surgical site. It presents as polyuria with a low urine osmolality despite normal/high serum osmolality. Treatment is by estimating and replacing the fluid deficit (which is hypo-osmolar) and the administration of desmopressin (DDAVP), a synthetic ADH analogue.

■ **CSF rhinorrhoea**
Generally no treatment is required although the risk of infection is probably increased. CSF drainage may reduce the pressure sufficiently to allow the leak to seal.

■ **Postoperative pain**

References
Smith M, Hirsch NP. Pituitary disease and anaesthesia. *BJA*, July 2000, Volume 85 (1), p3–14
Stone DJ *et al. The Neuroanaesthesia Handbook*, chapter 12 – Pituitary Surgery, p231–249. Mosby 1996, St Louis, Missouri, USA

Acute asthma   ✓

You are called to the accident and emergency department to see a 31-year-old lady, known to have asthma, who has been admitted with acute shortness of breath.

How would you make a clinical assessment of the severity of this attack?

> This is a common clinical scenario and therefore requires a punchy answer because you will have seen it frequently. Don't forget that before examining for specific physical signs, a brief history should be obtained if possible.

■ History   From patient/relative/paramedic
Speed of onset
Previous treatment
Previous attacks requiring artificial ventilation

Clinical features of **acute severe** asthma include:

■ Inability to complete sentences
■ Tachycardia > 110 beats/min
■ Respiratory rate > 25/min
■ PEFR < 50% of predicted or best

Clinical features of **life-threatening** asthma include:

- Silent chest
- Cyanosis
- Bradycardia
- Confusion
- Exhaustion
- PEFR < 33% of predicted or best

Other clinical signs of an acute asthma attack include **sweating, bounding pulse, wheeze** (which points to the diagnosis but may not be evident if there is a severe reduction in air flow) and **pulsus paradoxus** (a fall in systolic blood pressure on inspiration due to increased lung volume) which is both difficult to assess and unreliable. A patient may be too exhausted to generate any large swings in intrathoracic pressure to produce the pulsus paradoxus.

What investigations might be helpful?

Asthma is primarily a clinical diagnosis but further information may be gained from a few investigations.

- **Peak expiratory flow rate** – as outlined above
- **CXR** – performed to exclude a pneumothorax and may show pulmonary hyperinflation
- **Arterial blood gases** – initially these may show hypocarbia with some degree of hypoxia. As the acute attack progresses worrying results include a normal/high $PaCO_2$ and $PaO_2 < 8$ kPa. Some degree of metabolic acidosis is inevitable
- **ECG** – this invariably shows a tachycardia but may also reveal p-pulmonale, right axis deviation, arrhythmias and ST elevation

Apart from an acute exacerbation of asthma, what would you include in your differential diagnosis?

The two most common differential diagnoses in adults would probably be **left ventricular failure** and **chronic obstructive airways disease**.
  Others include:

- Pulmonary embolism
- Upper airway obstruction
- Inhaled foreign body
- Aspiration
- Churg–Strauss syndrome (allergic granulomatosis)
- Aspergillosis

What would be your immediate management of this lady?

- **Sit the patient up**
- **Oxygen**   As high a concentration as possible from a facemask (reservoir)

■ β_2 agonists   Starting with 2.5–5 mg of salbutamol nebulised in oxygen and repeated as required. If there is no response (or a deterioration) this may be given intravenously at a dose of 3–20 μg/min. It should be noted however that some investigators have concluded that intravenous β_2 agonists may be less effective than nebulised. Side-effects include tachycardia, arrhythmias, tremor, hyperglycaemia, hypokalaemia and lactic acidosis.

■ **Anticholinergics**   Nebulised in oxygen e.g. ipratropium bromide 0.5 mg. These agents seem to be synergistic with the β_2 agonists.

■ **Steroids**   The role of steroids in acute severe asthma is now well established and they should be given soon after presentation. Normal practice is to give 200 mg of intravenous hydrocortisone. Peak response is at 6–12 hours.

■ **Aminophylline**   This still remains a controversial area and is generally used in patients who have failed to respond to the above therapy. It is given intravenously as a loading dose of 3 mg/kg followed by an infusion of 0.5 mg/kg/h. The loading dose is omitted in patients who have been receiving oral theophyllines. Toxic side effects include arrhythmias and convulsions (> 40 mg/L) as well as nausea, vomiting, headache and restlessness.

■ **Fluids and electrolytes**   These patients will have both reduced intake and increased losses and careful fluid replacement is indicated. Hypokalaemia is relatively common.

■ **Regular reassessment**

What other less well-established treatments do you know about?

■ **Magnesium**   There are various theories about its mechanism of action:
- Ca^{2+} antagonist effect in bronchial smooth muscle
- High sympathetic activity can reduce Mg^{2+} levels
- Mg^{2+} reduces Ach release at the neuromuscular junction and may therefore reduce bronchospasm
- May increase sensitivity of β receptors to catecholamines in severe asthma

■ **Adrenaline**

■ **Ketamine**

■ **Inhalational agents**   These have bronchodilator effects but there is the risk of cardiovascular side effects

■ **Helium**   This reduces the work of breathing by reducing gas density and therefore turbulent flow

■ **Bronchoscopy and lavage**

■ **ECMO**

What are the indications for mechanical ventilation?

- Respiratory arrest
- Reducing level of consciousness or coma
- Exhaustion
- Increasing hypoxaemia despite maximal medical treatment
- Increasing acidosis despite maximal medical treatment

Mechanical ventilatory support is required in 1–3% of acute admissions with asthma.

What are the important points of the ventilator settings in asthmatics?

There are many changes in lung physiology which cause problems for mechanical ventilation:

- Airflow obstruction means lung overinflation is a hazard – risk of barotrauma/pneumothorax
- Lung units will have variably increased time constants so long inspiratory times may be necessary to provide time for adequate gas exchange. This is not as commonly appreciated as the need for long expiratory times
- Lung overinflation reduces venous return, compresses the heart and increases pulmonary vascular resistance

> The principles in ventilation are to limit peak and mean airway pressures, allow a prolonged expiratory time and maintain adequate oxygenation in the face of a high $PaCO_2$.

Strategies include:

- Low respiratory rate
- Low tidal volumes may be necessary to avoid barotrauma
- I:E ratio with prolonged expiratory time
- The use of extrinsic PEEP remains controversial
- Permissive hypercapnia

If it becomes impossible to ventilate the patient or there is a precipitous drop in cardiac output, the ventilator should be disconnected from the endotracheal tube and the lungs manually deflated by compression on the chest.

References

McConachie I. *Handbook of ICU Therapy*, 1999, p215–224. Greenwich Medical Media, London
Salmeron S, *et al*. Nebulised versus intravenous albuterol in hypercapnic acute asthma: a multicentre, double blind, randomised study. *Am J Respir Crit Care Med* 1994, Volume 149, p1466–1470

Airway assessment

How do you assess a patient's airway prior to anaesthesia?

Remember:

- History
- Examination
- Investigations

This is easy to forget in examination conditions

- **History**   Any history of previous problems with airway management must be elicited and the anaesthetic charts reviewed
- **Examination**
- **Anatomical problems**   Obesity
  Large breasts
  Prominent teeth
  Short, thick neck
  Syndromes associated with difficult intubation
  Trauma, local infection, radiotherapy
- **Mallampati score**   This assesses the visibility of the pharyngeal structures and assumes the view is related to the size of the tongue base. The further assumption is that a large tongue base may hinder exposure of the larynx. Initially there were 3 proposed classes, but Samsoon and Young added a fourth in 1987 and this has gained common acceptance

Mallampati score
Technique – patient sitting, head neutral, mouth fully open and tongue fully extended, no phonation. Some suggest conducting the test twice.

- Class I   Exposure of soft palate, uvula and tonsillar pillars
- Class II   Exposure of soft palate and base of uvula
- Class III Exposure of soft palate only
- Class IV   No visualisation of pharyngeal structures except hard palate

- **Forward mandibular movement**
- **Cervical spine movement**   Assesses atlanto-occipital and atlanto-axial joint mobility. The patient is asked to extend the head with the neck in full flexion
- **Thyromental distance**   Described in 1983 by Patil *et al* and defined as the distance from the chin to the notch of the thyroid cartilage with the head fully extended. If this is less than 6 cm, it may be associated with difficult intubation

■ **Sternomental distance**   Described in 1994 by Savva and defined as the distance from the tip of the chin to the sternal notch. If this is less than 12 cm, it may be associated with difficult intubation

■ **Prayer sign**   Difficult intubation has been associated with the inability to place both palms flat together and seems to be more common in diabetics

Wilson Risk Score

Wilson Risk Score
This gives a score from 0–2 for each of the following risk factors:

■ Weight
■ Head and neck movement
■ Jaw movement
■ Receding mandible
■ Buck teeth

A score of 3 or more predicts 75% of difficult intubations (with 12% incidence of false positives).

Individually, these tests have only moderate sensitivity and specificity. More recently, investigators have looked at combined predictors to try and increase the usefulness of these tests.

The combination of Mallampati class III/IV with a thyromental distance of less than 7 cm is predictive of a grade IV laryngoscopy with high sensitivity and specificity.

■ **Investigations**   Plain X-rays of head and neck
                        CT scan
                        Fibreoptic laryngoscopy

Some useful terms
Difficult intubation   When placement of an endotracheal tube requires more than three attempts and/or more than 10 mins (ASA, 1993)
Difficult laryngoscopy   As described by Cormack and Lehane
Difficult mask ventilation   Less clearly defined but certainly a different entity to the concepts above. One study showed a 15% incidence of difficult mask ventilation in patients who had difficult or failed intubation.

How would you manage a difficult airway?

A difficult airway may be recognised preoperatively as described above or may be unrecognised, presenting itself when the patient is anaesthetised and/or paralysed. These two situations warrant different management. The basic principles common to both include:

■ Call for experienced (in difficult airway) senior anaesthetic help
■ Call for experienced surgical help
■ Maintain oxygenation
■ Ensure difficult airway adjuncts are available
■ Have working knowledge of a difficult airway algorithm

Recognised difficult airway

With anticipated difficult airway management, the airway should be secured with the patient awake. Preparation in this case is essential. Consideration should be given to the following:

■ Psychological preparation of the patient
■ Monitoring
■ Drying agents
■ Aspiration prophylaxis
■ Sedation
■ Oxygen supplementation
■ Topical local anaesthesia +/– nerve blocks
■ Topical vasoconstrictors
■ Appropriate equipment

If intubation fails in these circumstances, options include:

1. Cancellation of surgery
2. Regional anaesthesia   It must be recognised that this could result in the need for general anaesthesia and airway control in suboptimal conditions should the regional block fail
3. Surgical airway

Unrecognised difficult airway

This presents a very different scenario and management depends on whether mask ventilation is possible or not.

If mask ventilation is possible, intubation choices range from various rigid laryngoscope blades, blind oral or nasal technique, fibreoptic, retrograde, illuminating stylet, rigid bronchoscope or percutaneous dilatational tracheostomy. Consideration must also be given to waking the patient up, a surgical airway or anaesthesia with mask ventilation.

If mask ventilation proves impossible ('cannot-ventilate, cannot-intubate' situation) a true emergency exists. There are now four possible options:

■ LMA
■ Combitube

- Transtracheal jet ventilation
- Surgical airway

It must be noted that the first two are supraglottic devices and may fail if the obstruction lies at or below the glottic opening.

References

Deakin CD. *Clinical Notes for the FRCA*, 1998, Churchill Livingstone, Edinburgh

Freck CM. Predicting difficult intubation. *Anaesthesia*, 1991, Volume 46, p1005–1008

Hagberg CA. *Handbook of Difficult Airway Management*, 2000. Churchill Livingstone, Philadelphia, USA

Amniotic fluid embolism

You are the anaesthetist on-call for delivery suite. You are called urgently to a delivery room where a woman in the second stage of labour has collapsed. Just prior to this she became extremely breathless and went blue, according to the midwife. She is now not breathing.

What is your immediate management?

> **Resuscitation** – this should be easy marks because it is 'bread and butter'.
>
> **Always** follow the ABC approach. You can be talking about this whilst thinking about the differential diagnosis.

- Call for **immediate help** from a senior obstetrician and anaesthetist
- If not breathing and no pulse – commence **CPR** and get defibrillator
- Establish an **airway** – the trachea should be intubated if appropriate
- Establish **breathing** with 100% oxygen
- **Circulation** – Large-bore intravenous cannulae should be sited with blood sent for crossmatch, coagulation screen, full blood count, urea, electrolytes and blood glucose
- Commence fluid resuscitation
- **Left lateral tilt**/Manual uterine displacement
- After 5 minutes consideration should be given to caesarian section to aid resuscitation attempts

There is no evidence of blood loss. What is the differential diagnosis?

The causes of sudden cardiovascular collapse in pregnancy are:

- **Amniotic fluid embolism**
- **Pulmonary thrombo-embolism**
- **Venous air embolism**

- **Occult haemorrhage** such as **placental abruption** or **hepatic rupture** in a patient with fulminating pre-eclampsia/HELLP
- **Intra-cerebral bleed**
- **Drug toxicity**
- **Sepsis**
- **Myocardial infarction**

What do you know about amniotic fluid embolism?

- Rare (1:20 000 deliveries) but devastating complication of labour or early puerperium
- Presents with **severe dyspnoea, cyanosis and sudden cardiovascular collapse** (with or without bleeding). **Seizures** may also occur
- **Cardiac arrest** occurs in up to 87%
- Up to 50% die in the first hour and the overall mortality is in the order of 85%
- Permanent brain damage is common in the survivors
- Amniotic fluid contains foetal debris, prostaglandins and leukotrienes which block pulmonary vessels, cause pulmonary vasoconstriction and lead to complement activation
- The US national registry concluded that the **pathophysiology was more in-keeping with an anaphylactoid reaction** rather than purely an embolic process as foetal squames have been found in the lungs of women without AFE syndrome
- Three major factors contribute to the problems encountered in this condition:

  1. **Acute pulmonary embolism**
  2. **Disseminated intravascular coagulation (DIC)**
  3. **Uterine atony**

- **Extreme hypoxia** is caused by lung and heart shunts
  Lung shunt   The transient increase in PVR may cause a shift of blood flow from blocked pulmonary vessels to patent ones resulting in incomplete oxygenation as the blood-flow through them overwhelms the maximum rate of oxygenation.
     The fall in cardiac output results in a fall in mixed venous O_2 saturation returning to the heart compounding oxygenation problems.
     There may be direct myocardial depression with pulmonary oedema.
  Heart shunt   A (potentially) patent foramen ovale is present in 35% of the population. Very high PA pressures may cause mixed venous blood to pass through it.
- **Severe left-sided heart failure** (mechanism unclear) causes hypotension
- **Coagulopathy** (in up to 83%) is probably caused by tissue factor or trophoblasts in the amniotic fluid stimulating the clotting cascade
- **Diagnosis** is based on clinical presentation and laboratory findings. Monoclonal antibody TKH-2 has been used to demonstrate foetal mucin in the pulmonary vasculature but it may still not be specific for the syndrome.

How would you manage this lady after delivery of the foetus?

- Intensive care
- Survivors of the initial event are at risk of: ARDS
                                                    Heart failure
                                                    DIC
- Treatment is supportive: Ventilation
                                                    Inotropic support
                                                    Clotting factors
- Uterine atony may necessitate oxytocin and carboprost (Hemabate™) (PGF$_2$)
- No form of therapy has been found to improve outcome
- Hydrocortisone and adrenaline have been recommended due to the similarity of the condition with anaphylaxis

References

Locksmith GJ. Amniotic fluid embolism. *Obstetrics and Gynaecology Clinics of North America* 1999, Volume 26(3), p435–444

Martin RW. Amniotic fluid embolism. *Clinical Obstetrics and Gynaecology* 1996, Volume 39(1), p101–106

Noble WH, St-Amand J. Amniotic fluid embolus. *Canadian Journal of Anaesthesia* 1993, Volume 40(10), p971–980

Oh TE. *Intensive Care Manual, 4th edition*, 1997. BH publishing, Oxford

Analgesia for circumcision ✓

I want you to imagine I am the mother of a 2-year-old boy due to come into hospital for circumcision. I am very worried that he will suffer with pain after the operation.

Can you explain to me how you will prevent this?

> This is a 'fluffy jumper' question that can easily be tackled badly! However, you should try to role-play and act in an interested and compassionate way! Your explanation should be in layman's terms.

'I can appreciate your concern. We tend to use a combination of techniques for pain relief, which keep the children comfortable after the operation. The first thing we will do, once he is asleep, is to put an injection of **local anaesthetic** into the base of his penis. This usually provides good pain relief for up to 12 hours after the operation. In addition to this we have a variety of other pain relief options available. We would start with simple **paracetamol** followed by the addition of something stronger like **brufen** or **voltarol**. Local **anaesthetic gel** (lignocaine) can also be smeared onto the wound regularly to cover the first 24–36 hours. These measures provide good pain relief and can be administered by you at home. It can be a bit sore at home for a few days but the medicines I have mentioned will keep him comfortable. In the rare event that something stronger was needed we might use **morphine liquid** to drink but we would keep him in hospital if that were the case.'

How can you assess post-operative pain in children?

An assessment of pain can be made by experienced staff with the use of routine monitoring (**HR, BP** and **respiratory rate**) together with **behavioural assessment techniques** (e.g. child withdrawn or lashing out). It is important to repeat the assessments and **listen to the parents**. In older children (>4 years) one can use **numerical pain-rating scales** or **visual scales** like the face self-reporting scale providing they have been understood pre-operatively.

What is the nerve supply to the penis?

The nerve supply to the penis is derived from the **pudendal nerve** (S2–4) which gives off the **dorsal nerve of the penis** bilaterally. These run **deep to Buck's fascia** and are just lateral to the dorsal arteries and veins bilaterally. They supply the distal two thirds of the penis. Ventral branches from the dorsal nerves supply the frenulum. The **genitofemoral and ilioinguinal nerves** may also provide some sensory supply at the base.

Once the child is asleep and being monitored by a second anaesthetist, how do you perform a penile block?

The dorsal nerves are blocked with injections of **0.5% plain bupivacaine** either side of the midline deep to Buck's fascia. The volume would be **1 ml + 0.1 ml/kg**. This ensures that the local anaesthetic passes posteriorly to block the ventral branches supplying the frenulum. **Bilateral blocks are necessary** because there is a midline septum, which may prevent spread from a single injection. The risk of vascular injury is also reduced.

Could you use a caudal?

Yes.

To estimate the volume and dose required the **regimen of Armitage** may be employed. Using 0.25% plain bupivacaine the volume is based on the weight and the level to be blocked.

- Lumbo-sacral block up to L1 – 0.5 ml/kg
- Block up to T10 – 1 ml/kg
- Block up to T6 – 1.25 ml/kg

What problems might be associated with a caudal?

- Dural tap
- Failure
- intravenous. injection
- Hypotension (rare in children)

- Urinary retention
- Motor weakness necessitating overnight stay in hospital

References

Brown TCK, Eyres RL, McDougall RJ. Local and regional anaesthesia in children. *BJA*, July 1999, Volume 83, p65–77

Mather SJ, Hughes DG. *A Handbook of Paediatric Anaesthesia*, 2nd edition, 1996. Oxford University Press, Oxford

Anaphylaxis ✓

You are anaesthetising a young woman for a hysteroscopy. Shortly following the injection of thiopentone, her blood pressure becomes unrecordable, she is flushed and her lungs are very difficult to ventilate with a bag and mask.

What are your <u>immediate</u> *actions?*

> You should be grinning inside if you get this question! The anaphylaxis drill should require practically no thought.

Anaphylaxis drill: *Initial therapy*

- **Stop administration** of suspected agent
- **Maintain airway: give 100% oxygen**
- **Lay the patient flat** with feet elevated
- **Give adrenaline:** **i.m.** at a dose of 0.5–1 mg (repeated every 10 mins if required)

  i.v. at a dose of 50–100 μg for hypotension or cardiovascular collapse titrated up to 0.5–1 mg as required
- **Give i.v. fluids** (crystalloid or colloid)

What secondary therapies would you administer or consider?

- **Antihistamines** – give chlorpheniramine 10–20 mg by slow i.v. infusion
- **Corticosteroids** – give hydrocortisone 100–300 mg i.v.
- **Catecholamine infusion**
- **Bronchodilators**
- **Consider bicarbonate (0.5–1 mmol/kg)**

How would you investigate this patient for suspected anaphylaxis?

Investigation can be divided into **immediate** and **late**. The diagnosis of anaphylactic or an anaphylactoid reaction hinges around the plasma tryptase concentration.

Immediate

Identification of an anaphylactic/anaphylactoid reaction:

➡ 1 hour after start of reaction   Take **10 ml venous blood** into a glass bottle
Separate serum and **store at –20°C**
Send to reference lab for **tryptase estimation**

Later

Identification of suspected agent.

- Skin prick tests
- Anaesthetist is responsible for ensuring they are performed (either by himself or, ideally, a specialist in interpretation of skin tests)

Tell me about plasma tryptase.

- Protein contained in mast cells – 99% of total body tryptase is within mast cells
- Released (along with histamine and other amines) in anaphylactic/anaphylactoid reactions
- **Sensitive and specific** diagnostic test for anaphylactic/anaphylactoid reactions
- Peak concentration at 1 h (concentration raised between 1 and 6 hours following mast-cell degranulation)
- Half-life 2.5 h
- Basal level = 0.8–1.5 ng/ml
- **Level >20 ng/ml seen in anaphylactic reactions**

NB   Urinary methylhistamine is the principal metabolite of histamine but is difficult to interpret outside the normal range although it will be detectable for longer than plasma tryptase.

How do you perform skin prick tests?

- Testing should include a wide range of anaesthetic drugs as well as the suspected agents to establish those drugs that are safe for future use
- Performed with 'neat' drug and 1 in 10 dilution
- Positive control (histamine) and negative control (phenol saline) should be included for each test
- A drop of drug is applied to the volar aspect of the forearm and a lancet stabbed through it to break the skin but not draw blood
- Sites are inspected over 15 minutes for weal and flare
- A weal of >2 mm larger than the negative control is regarded as positive
- **A positive skin-prick test to 1 in 10 solution is a true positive** (true reactions may have positive tests at much greater dilutions e.g. 1 in 100 or 1 in 1000)
- A positive test to 'neat' drug may or may not be significant

> **Reporting:**
> ■ Full explanation to the patient (Medic-alert braclet)
> ■ Record in the case notes
> ■ Inform GP
> ■ Report to the Committee on the Safety of Medicines

Reference

Suspected Anaphylactic Reactions Associated with Anaesthesia, 1995, revised edition. Published by the Association of Anaesthetists of Great Britain and Ireland and The British Society of Allergy and Clinical Immunology (working party).

Antepartum haemorrhage ✓

You are called to the labour ward to see a 25-year-old P_{2+1} lady in labour who has lost 700 ml of blood PV in labour. She looks pale and sweaty, her pulse is 140, regular and thready and her BP is 105/55.

What would you do?

■ **ABC**
■ Administer 100% oxygen via a non-rebreathing reservoir face-mask
■ Establish intravenous access with two large-bore cannulae
■ Commence fluid resuscitation with crystalloid/colloid (not dextrans)
■ O-negative blood initially (usually 2 units available on the ward) until group-specific/fully cross-matched blood available (group-specific takes 15 minutes)
■ Pressure bags and fluid warmer
■ Head-down, left lateral tilt
■ Call obstetrician, midwives and another anaesthetist (consultant if possible)
■ Inform haematologist
■ Send blood for FBC, crossmatch at least 6 units, coagulation screen, urea, electrolytes and LFTs
■ Regular repeated Hb, platelet and coagulation studies
■ Consider FFP, cryoprecipitate and platelets
■ There may be a major haemorrhage trolley on the delivery suite
■ Joint assessment with obstetricians as to the urgency of surgery
■ Adequate maternal monitoring (CVP and invasive BP useful if there is time)
■ Foetal monitoring
■ Treat the cause

How would you assess the degree of blood loss?

The losses into the bed and onto pads could be estimated and the degree of hypovolaemia estimated by using physical signs such as tachycardia, BP, capillary refill time, skin colour and level of consciousness.

There may be an underestimation of the degree of hypovolaemia due to hidden losses.

What are the likely causes of her bleeding?

- Placenta praevia ⎫ Most
- Placental abruption ⎬ likely
- Uterine rupture
- Cervical or vaginal tear
- Uterine atony
- Coagulation or platelet problem

Her previous pregnancy resulted in a caesarian section. Is this relevant?

Yes. This increases the possibility of **placenta praevia** overlying the old uterine scar and increases the risk of uterine rupture. There is also a higher incidence of placenta accreta (adheres to the surface), increta (invades uterine muscle) or percreta (penetrates through uterine muscle) all of which may lead to life-threatening haemorrhage necessitating a hysterectomy to stop the bleeding.

How would you anaesthetise this lady?

- Initial resuscitation as already outlined
- Aspiration prophylaxis
- Rapid sequence induction with cricoid pressure and left lateral tilt on the operating table
- Equipment for a difficult intubation should be available
- Consultant anaesthetist ideally in attendance or at least two pairs of 'anaesthetic hands'

What measures are available to influence the degree of blood loss on the table?

These can be divided into surgical, medical and haematological:

Surgical	Bimanual uterine compression and packing
	Aortic compression
	Uterine or internal iliac artery ligation
	Hysterectomy
	Arterial embolisation
Medical	Keep anaesthetic vapour concentration down
	Ergometrine
	Oxytocin
	Carboprost (Hemabate™) – PGF$_{2\alpha}$
Haematological	FFP
	Cryoprecipitate
	Platelets

References

Goldstone JC, Pollard BJ. *Handbook of Clinical Anaesthesia*, 1996. Churchill Livingstone, Edinburgh

Oh TE. *Intensive Care Manual* 1997. Butterworth-Heinemann, Oxford

Revised Guidelines for the Management of Massive Obstetric Haemorrhage, 1994. Report on Confidential Enquiry into Maternal Deaths in the UK

Awareness

You are called to see a patient on the surgical ward by the Sister because the patient describes being aware during surgery (you did not anaesthetise the patient).

How do you deal with the situation?

■ **Inform the anaesthetist involved** and the head of the department – there may be a departmental policy or someone with a special interest in awareness

■ Interview the patient with a senior colleague – (ideally the anaesthetist involved should do this). Always have a witness present

■ Establish the events surrounding the time of alleged awareness by reviewing the anaesthetic charts, discussing with the anaesthetist involved and the patient

■ Establish whether it is true recall or dreaming. Recall may be further divided into explicit (patient can recall conversations which took place in theatre) or implicit (behavioural changes post-operatively due to intra-operative subconscious learning)

■ Establish whether the patient was in pain – this has implications for long-term psychological sequelae such as nightmares and flashbacks

■ If there was a clear lapse in the standard of anaesthetic care then honesty with an admission of fault and an apology is appropriate

■ Document all conversations and assessments in the case notes

■ Hospital management including the legal department may need to be informed in order that the events can be documented for future reference in case of legal action

■ Offer counselling for the patient

What do you tell the patient?

It is important to acknowledge the patient's feelings and let them know you believe what they are saying. This helps with the well-recognised psychological sequelae following an episode of awareness. These include anxiety, insomnia, nightmares, depression, a morbid fear of hospitals and doctors and a preoccupation with death. It is helpful to explain why awareness might have occurred: through no particular fault but instead because of the need to minimise the doses of anaesthetic agents given. If there is clear fault on the part of the anaesthetist then it may still be wise to admit it. Although this is an admission of negligence some say it may help to reduce anxiety for future anaesthetics if there was a definite reason for the awareness.

In summary, a full explanation of the events and an apology are recommended.

What is the legal situation regarding awareness?

An anaesthetist has a duty of care towards a patient. A patient who is going to have a general anaesthetic expects to be asleep and unaware. To decide whether there is a breach in the duty of care the **Bolam test** is applied.

In the 1950s Bolam's leg was broken during a course of ECT. Bolam's expert witnesses claimed that the omission of a muscle relaxant was negligent. The experts called by the hospital were of the opinion that muscle relaxants were not essential. The judge ruled that:

> 'A doctor is not guilty of negligence if acting in accordance with a practice accepted as proper by a responsible body of medical opinion even though a body of adverse opinion also exists amongst medical men.'

An anaesthetist must therefore prove that the technique he used is one that is considered to be reasonable by his peers. This is done through review of the anaesthetic records by expert witnesses. If there is evidence of a shortfall in the standard of anaesthetic care then the anaesthetist is guilty of negligence.

If the awareness can be clearly linked to the poor anaesthetic technique ('causation') then compensation is payable.

When is awareness most likely?

- At induction and intubation
- On transfer from the anaesthetic room to theatre
- During procedures involving the use of muscle relaxants
- TIVA
- During procedures where low concentrations of volatile are used deliberately e.g. LSCS or hypotensive patient
- At emergence

Awareness with explicit recall has a reported incidence of approximately 1/500 and is most common during obstetric GA (especially at intubation). Awareness with pain is far less common.

What are the causes of awareness?

- **Induction**   Low doses of drugs as above
                     Intubation too early or delayed due to difficulty or
                     waiting for relaxant to work
- **Transfer**   Induction agent levels fall before adequate partial
                     pressure of volatile builds up

■ **During surgery**　Equipment failure, e.g. breathing system leak/disconnection, vaporiser malfunction or exhaustion, TIVA line tissued

How do you monitor depth of anaesthesia?

■ **Simple clinical signs**	BP, HR, sweating, lacrimation, pupils
■ **MAC**	Based on population studies
■ **Isolated forearm technique**	
■ **Spontaneous skeletal muscle activity**	Frontalis, lost with relaxants
■ **Oesophageal contractility**	Depth of anaesthesia related to frequency of contractions
■ **Evoked potentials**	Visual, auditory, somatosensory (changes in latency and amplitude)
■ **EEG**	
■ **Spectral edge frequency**	Frequency when significant EEG activity is seen
■ **Cerebral function monitor**	Processed EEG makes interpretation easier
■ **Bispectral index**	
■ **Heart rate variability**	'Fathom' monitor – loss of respiratory sinus arrhythmia

---

Guedel Classification of the Stages of Anaesthesia (Described in 1937, spontaneous respiration with ether)

■ **Stage 1**　**Analgesia**　　Start of induction to LOC
　　　　　　　　　　　　　　Regular, small volume respiration
　　　　　　　　　　　　　　Normal pupils

■ **Stage 2**　**Excitement**　　LOC to onset of automatic breathing
　　　　　　　　　　　　　　Irregular respiration
　　　　　　　　　　　　　　Dilated, divergent pupils
　　　　　　　　　　　　　　Active airway reflexes
　　　　　　　　　　　　　　Loss of eyelash reflex

■ **Stage 3**　**Surgical anaesthesia**
　　　　　　　　Plane 1: Regular, large volume respiration
　　　　　　　　　　　　Eye movements stop, pinpoint pupils
　　　　　　　　　　　　Loss of eyelid reflex
　　　　　　　　Plane 2: Intercostal respiration reduced
　　　　　　　　　　　　Loss of corneal reflex
　　　　　　　　Plane 3: Diaphragmatic respiration
　　　　　　　　　　　　Laryngeal reflexes reduced
　　　　　　　　Plane 4: Diaphragmatic respiration reduced
　　　　　　　　　　　　Carinal reflex depressed
　　　　　　　　　　　　Dilated pupils

■ **Stage 4**　**Coma**　　　　Apnoea, hypotension

A

References

Aitkinhead AR. Awareness during anaesthesia: what should the patient be told? *Anaesthesia*, 1990, Volume 45, p351–352

Aitkinhead AR. The pattern of litigation against anaesthetists. *BJA*, 1994, Volume 73, p10–21

Aitkinhead AR, Smith G. *Textbook of Anaesthesia, third edition* 1996, p403–4. Churchill Livingstone, Edinburgh

Craft T, Upton P. *Key topics in Anaesthesia, 2nd edition* 1995. Bios Scientific Publications, Oxford

Dealing with Negligence Claims. Medical Protection Society publication

Deakin CD. *Clinical Notes for the FRCA*. 1998 Churchill Livingstone

Pomfrett CJD. Awareness. *Handbook of Clinical Anaesthesia* 1996, p614–615. Churchill Livingstone

Pomfrett CJD. Monitoring depth of anaesthesia. November 2000, Bulletin 4, The Royal College of Anaesthetists

Bends ✓

You are an anaesthetist in a seaside town and are asked to assess a 22-year-old man who has been scuba diving and brought into the accident department unconscious.

How would you manage this patient initially?

The initial management would be generalised as the diagnosis is not known at this stage. Any history of preceding events may direct further therapy at the most likely diagnosis:

- Airway   Attention should be given to the possibility of a head or neck injury and the C-spine immobilised
- Breathing   Highest FiO_2 available
- Circulation   Large bore cannulae and fluids

Can you list some differential diagnoses?

- Decompression sickness
- Near-drowning
- Head injury
- Convulsion – oxygen induced
- Hypoxia
- Hypothermia
- Coincidental pathology e.g. intracranial haemorrhage/cerebral infarction

What is decompression sickness?

Decompression 'illness' may be described in terms of two syndromes:

1. Decompression sickness
2. Pulmonary barotrauma and arterial gas embolism

Decompression sickness

During a dive the increased ambient pressure causes nitrogen to dissolve into tissues.

On ascent the decrease in pressure causes the nitrogen that has been dissolved in the body tissues to come out of solution. If ascent is too rapid then the partial pressure of nitrogen in the tissues will rise above tissue hydrostatic pressure and gas bubbles form. Symptoms range from pains in the tissues around joints (the classical **'bends'**) to neurological impairment such as visual disturbances, convulsions, paraparesis and loss of consciousness. Nitrogen bubbles may also migrate from tissues into the venous system to cause **venous gas embolism**. This is usually asymptomatic. However, high levels of venous gas embolism in the pulmonary circulation can cause pulmonary hypertension, pulmonary oedema, retrosternal discomfort, cough and dyspnoea ('**the chokes**').

Pulmonary barotrauma and arterial gas embolism

Pulmonary barotrauma results from a diver holding his breath during ascent. This may cause pneumothorax, pneumomediastinum or arterial gas embolism.

Arterial bubbles occlude vessels after which platelets and fibrin may be deposited at the bubble–blood interface. There may also be bubble–endothelium interactions culminating in a delayed reduction in blood flow and capillary leak.

Note that pulmonary barotrauma and arterial gas embolism may occur after a breath-hold dive of only one metre whereas decompression sickness requires a significant depth–time exposure.

How is it treated?

■ **Fluids ABC**	Immersion diuresis and bubble-induced endothelial damage may result in severe dehydration. Aggressive fluid administration may also improve the rate of nitrogen washout. Use isotonic fluids without glucose
■ **Oxygen**	Improves delivery to underperfused tissues but also reduces the partial pressure of nitrogen in the blood and hence in the tissues surrounding the bubble. The increase in tissue–bubble partial pressure gradient facilitates diffusion of nitrogen from the bubble back into the tissues thus shrinking it and reducing symptoms
■ **Recompression**	The idea is to force gas back into solution initially and then allow excretion at a more controlled rate. A commonly used treatment table is that used by the US Navy. It consists of recompression at 25 ft/min to a depth of 60 ft (2.8 atm) followed by hyperbaric oxygen therapy at two depths – 60 ft and 30 ft. The rate of ascent is typically 1 ft/min and the length of treatment is variable depending on the depth and length of dive. The inspired pressure of oxygen should not be greater than 3 atmospheres and is given typically in cycles of 20 minutes separated by breathing air for 5–15 minutes. If airborne transfer is required the patient is transferred with 100% oxygen at sea-level cabin pressure.
■ **Position**	Supine Head-down position has no proven role in preventing arterial bubbles entering the cerebral circulation and may increase cerebral oedema. There is similarly no benefit in massive venous gas embolism. Therefore, the head-down position is not routinely recommended except perhaps in severe hypotension. However, placing the injured diver in the supine position has two advantages. It may help to prevent hypotension and the rate of nitrogen washout is greater than in the sitting position.

■ **Avoid hyperglycaemia**
■ **Avoid hyperthermia**

Reference

Moon RE. Treatment of diving emergencies. *Critical Care Clinics*, April 1999, Volume 15, Number 2, p429–456

Bleeding tonsil

You are called to see a 4-year-old boy on the paediatric ward. He had a tonsillectomy 4 hours previously and has been vomiting blood for the last hour. His heart rate is 150 and his blood pressure is 95/60.

What are the problems in managing this case?

Problems:
- **Frightened child** and anxious parents
- **Hypovolaemia**
- **Full stomach**
- **Residual effects of the anaesthetic** 4 hours earlier
- **Difficult intubation** – bleeding and possible upper airway oedema from the previous intubation and surgery

Review of the previous anaesthetic chart and history and examination are, of course, mandatory. The consultant anaesthetist should be informed.

It is vital to ensure he is adequately resuscitated before embarking on another anaesthetic. Intravenous access should be established and resuscitation commenced with crystalloid/colloid 20 ml/kg (APLS recommends crystalloid).

How would you estimate blood loss?

The most helpful indicators of hypovolaemia are:

- **Heart rate**
- **Pulse volume**
- **Capillary-refill time** (pressure for 5 s then release, normal refill < 2 s)
- **Skin colour** (mottling/pallor/peripheral cyanosis)
- **Blood pressure** (80 + (2 x age in years); hypotension is a late sign
- **Conscious level**

The **degree of blood loss is often underestimated**. Looking at the amount of blood vomited will be inaccurate because much of it is likely to have been swallowed. Haemoglobin and haematocrit estimations may help. Postural hypotension suggests significant hypovolaemia but measuring this would not be practical in a frightened child. Core:peripheral temperature difference >2°C is a sign of poor perfusion to skin. Respiratory rate may be high as a compensatory response to hypovolaemic metabolic acidosis. He should have blood cross-matched and available in theatre.

What anaesthetic technique would you employ?

There are two schools of thought as to the method of induction:

- **Rapid sequence induction** with cricoid pressure
- **Gas induction** in the head-down, left lateral position

A **rapid sequence induction with cricoid pressure** in the supine position is likely to be the most familiar technique. Although it is recognised that cricoid pressure does not protect the airway from bleeding in the pharynx, it is the technique most likely to secure the airway quickly. (A gas induction in the head-down, left lateral position may be fraught with potential problems.) There should be **two suction devices** in case one becomes blocked with clot and a variety of tube sizes and laryngoscope blades. The **ENT surgeon needs to be scrubbed** and prepared to perform a tracheostomy should the need arise.

Following intubation, a **nasogastric tube** may be inserted to empty the stomach. This is then removed prior to extubation. Once haemostasis is achieved, the child is extubated awake and in the head-down, left-lateral position.

References

Deakin CD. *Clinical Notes for the FRCA*, 1998. Churchill Livingstone, Edinburgh

Mather SJ, Hughes DG. *A Handbook of Paediatric Anaesthesia*, 2nd edition 1996. Oxford University Press, Oxford

Burns ✓

A 35-year-old man is brought into the accident department having been rescued from a house-fire. He has burns to his face, arms and trunk but does not seem to be in much pain.

How would you assess the severity of the burn?

This can be assessed in several ways:

■ **Age** and **% of body surface area burnt** (using the rule of 9's) are the two most important prognostic factors

As a guide: **% mortality = BSA of burn + age**
Other factors influencing outcome (and therefore classifying the burn as more severe) are:

Associated inhalational injury (doubles mortality rate)
Coexistent medical problems

■ **Classified according to depth**

1°/Superficial	Epidermis
2°/Partial thickness	
Superficial	Outer dermis
	Capillary refill
	Painful
Deep	Some deep dermal damage
	Painless
	White
3°/Full thickness	Dermis destroyed
	Needs grafting

■ Using the **rule of 9's** the burn can be assessed as a **major burn** if:
    Full thickness burn >10% TBSA (Total Body Surface Area)
    Partial thickness burn >25% TBSA (or 20% at extremes of age)
    Burns to hands, feet or perineum
    Inhalational, chemical or electrical burns
    Burns in patients with serious pre-existing medical conditions

    Severe burn is >40% TBSA

How would you initially treat this patient?

Resuscitate the patient according to the ATLS guidelines:

■ **Airway**   Administer **100% oxygen** via a reservoir mask; this would also help to treat any CO poisoning. The **upper airway** is particularly susceptible to **oedema** and subsequent **obstruction**. A high index of suspicion should be maintained with regard to inhalational injury and **early intubation** with an **uncut tube** is frequently needed. **Suxamethonium** can be used in the first 24 hours. It should then be avoided for 2 years because the increased number of post-junctional receptors causes prolonged depolarisation and marked release of potassium.

■ **Breathing**   Blood gases should be taken immediately while remembering that the arterial PO_2 is unreliable for predicting CO poisoning. Early **bronchoscopy** if there is a risk of inhalational injury. If there is evidence of this injury then perform **broncho-alveolar lavage** with 20 ml aliquots of **1.4% bicarbonate** until the aspirate is clear. This should be followed by 10 ml instilled via the ET tube and 10 ml nebulised every hour until clear for 6 hours.

■ **Circulation**   **2 large bore i.v. cannulae** should be sited. These may be difficult to place and may need to be placed through a burn. Evaluation of **volume status** and use of a blood pressure cuff may be difficult in a burned patient. A **urinary catheter** and possibly an **arterial line** will be needed. One should aim for a urine output of at least 50 ml/hour in this patient.

Early referral to a regional burns centre would be appropriate.

How would you guide your fluid management?

There are several **formulae** that can help guide fluid management. Amongst them are:

Parkland	CSL 4 ml/kg/%TBSA in 24 hours (first half given in 8 hours)
Muir and Barclay (Mount Vernon)	0.5 ml PPF/albumin/kg/%TBSA every 4 hours for 12 hours, then 6 hourly for 12 hours
Brook	0.5 ml colloid/kg + 1.5 ml crystalloid/%TBSA, half over first 8 hours

The time of injury is the starting point for these calculations. It should be emphasised that these are only a **guide** and that assessment of resuscitation should be based clinically on **heart rate, BP, capillary refill, CVP, urine output**, peripheral and core **temperature** and the **mental state** of the patient. However, a PAFC is used in many centres as there is evidence of poor correlation between simple clinical parameters (heart rate and urine output) and the haemodynamics in severe burns.

What would make you suspicious of an inhalation injury?

- Points in the history:
  - Explosion
  - Fire in an enclosed space
  - Inhalation of toxic fumes
  - Alcohol intoxication
- On examination:
  - Burnt face
  - Raised carboxyhaemoglobin levels
  - Stridor
  - Soot in the sputum
  - Burnt eyebrows or nasal hair
  - Respiratory distress

Is pain management a problem with burns patients?

Yes. Apart from the initial injury they are subjected to multiple dressing changes and various operations. They develop **tolerance to opioids** very rapidly and therefore may require large doses of opioids and the use of **ketamine, entonox, paracetamol** and also **antidepressants**.

Other problems you could be asked about:

Early feeding	High catabolic state. Establishing N/G feeding in the first 4 hours improves outcome
Heat loss	Impaired homeostatic control and heat loss through burns
Sepsis	Impaired immune function
ARDS	Effects of burn wound mediators/plasma oncotic pressure/PAP. Multiple organ failure
Resistance to NMBs	May last 18 months (Ach receptors)
Arrhythmias and rhabdomyolysis	Occur with electrical burns
Burn wound excision	Limit to 20% per operation (warm theatre 28–32°C/ big drips/warm fluids/potential for large blood loss)
Haematological effects	↑ Hct for 48 hours – unreliable measure of resuscitation. ↓ rbc $t_{1/2}$. ↓ Platelets due to microaggregation. Degree of consumption coagulopathy. DIC possible. Later thrombogenicity (↓ Protein C, S and anti-Th III) → PE

References

Haji-Michael P. *Intensive Care Unit Guidelines for the Care of the Patient with Burns* (Version III, 8/99). Withington Hospital ICU, Manchester

MacLennan N, Heimbach DM, Cullen MD. Anaesthesia for major thermal injury. *Anesthesiology* Sept 1998, Volume 89, p749–770

Morgan GE, Mikhail MS. *Clinical Anaesthesiology*, 2nd edition, 1996. Appleton and Lange, Stamford, CT

Carbon monoxide poisoning

You are asked to see a male patient who has been found in his garage with the engine of his car running. His face is cherry red.

What is the likely diagnosis?

The patient is likely to be suffering from **carbon monoxide poisoning**. It must not be forgotten that there could be coexistent problems such as self-poisoning with tablets.

What is carbon monoxide poisoning?

The usual definition is a **level of greater than 20% carboxyhaemoglobin** in the blood. Co-oximetry is needed to make the diagnosis.
Symptoms are:

- **20–30%** Throbbing headache
  Irritability
  Fatiguability
  Poor judgement
  Nausea and vomiting
- **30–40%** Confusion
  Syncope on exertion
- **>50%** Coma
  Convulsions
  Death

How does carbon monoxide poisoning affect O_2 delivery at tissue level?

CO and O_2 both bind to the α-chain of the haemoglobin molecule, but CO has about 250 times the affinity for the ferrous iron complex compared with O_2. This is a competitive and reversible effect.
Tissue oxygen delivery is affected in 2 ways:

1. There is a reduction in the availability of oxygen-binding sites and therefore a **reduction in oxygen carrying capacity**.
2. CO interacts with the remaining haemoglobin molecule to increase the affinity for the oxygen it carries. This results in a **left shift of the oxyhaemoglobin dissociation curve** such that haemoglobin is less keen to give up oxygen at tissue level. Thus, oxygen delivery is further reduced.

How would you manage carbon monoxide poisoning?

Resuscitation should always follow the ABC approach. The primary objective is to reverse tissue hypoxia. Removal of CO is of secondary importance. Oxygen is the treatment that accomplishes both of these goals. The patient should be given 100% oxygen. In severe cases hyperbaric oxygen therapy has been used (but is still controversial). Hyperbaric oxygen therapy (HBO) can provide nearly all the body's oxygen needs purely from the dissolved oxygen.

Poor prognostic indicators are:

- Increased duration of exposure
- Increasing age
- Low GCS at time of admission

Current criteria for HBO therapy are:
- Carboxyhaemoglobin > 20%
- Loss of consciousness at any stage
- Neurological signs and symptoms (except headache)
- Myocardial ischaemia/arrhythmia
- Pregnancy

Coexistent problems such as other forms of self-poisoning or burns should also be addressed. The decision to transfer a patient to a hyperbaric chamber (usually in a different hospital) must take into account the carboxyhaemoglobin level, the time needed to transfer the patient and the patient's fitness for transfer.

What is the half-life of COHb in air, 100% O_2 and hyperbaric O_2?

Air (21% O_2)	240–300 minutes
100% O_2 (1 atm)	40–80 minutes
100% O_2 (3 atm)	23–25 minutes

As can be seen from these figures, simply administering 100% oxygen will significantly expedite the removal of carbon monoxide.

References

Brenner BE. *Comprehensive Management of Respiratory Emergencies*. Aspen Systems Corp, 1995, USA

Hawkins M, Harrison J, Charters P. Severe carbon monoxide poisoning: outcome after hyperbaric oxygen therapy. *BJA* May 2000 ,Volume 84(5), p584–586

Cervical spine injury

What are the problems of anaesthetising a patient with a C6 transection 6 weeks after the accident?

Airway and breathing

Cervical spine	Difficult intubation – metalwork, reduced neck movement
Respiratory insufficiency	History of ICU admission
	Lower RTIs
	Impaired ability to cough
	Tracheostomy
	Atelectasis and V/Q mismatch

Circulation

■ Cardiovascular problems	**Autonomic hyperreflexia** **Postural hypotension** (may need preloading prior to induction) **Bradycardia** (especially with intubation, pretreat with atropine)
■ Venous access	Cannulation can be difficult with decreased skin blood flow
■ Anaemia	Especially with chronic sepsis

Renal

■ Renal impairment	Due to recurrent UTIs (catheters and vesico-ureteric reflux)

Drugs

■ Altered response to drugs	**Suxamethonium** – denervation hypersensitivity Receptors spread from the end-plate to cover the whole muscle. Avoid between 3 days and 9 months Decreased blood volume and decreased lean tissue mass result in decreased volumes of distribution for many drugs
■ Medication	Anticoagulants, dantrolene, baclofen

Other

■ Positioning intraoperatively	Pressure sores, contractures and spasms
■ Decreased gastric emptying	Risk of aspiration
■ Temperature	Patients can become partially poikilothermic as normal mechanisms of thermoregulation are impaired
■ Chronic pain problems	

Tell me about autonomic hyperreflexia.

- It is characterised by a grossly disordered autonomic response to certain stimuli below the level of the lesion
- Occurs in about 85% of patients with a lesion higher than T7
- Onset is from 3 weeks to 12 years post injury
- Results in hypertension (may be severe with diastolic >170 mmHg), sweating and headache. Reflex bradycardia and skin changes (pallor or flushing) above the level of the lesion are common
- Neurophysiologically there is loss of descending inhibition from higher centres and deranged alterations in connections within the distal spinal cord. This results in inappropriate sympathetic reflexes causing profound vasoconstriction

What are the triggers of autonomic hyperreflexia?

- Pelvic visceral stimulation (especially bladder distension) is very commonly implicated
- Bowel distension (including constipation)
- Uterine contractions
- Urinary tract infections
- Pressure sores

How is it treated?

- Removal of the cause (exclude bladder distension)
- Sit upright
- Drugs need to be of rapid onset: Sublingual nifedipine 10 mg
  GTN
  α-adrenergic blocking agents
  Hydralazine
  Clonidine
  Increasing depth of general anaesthesia
- Use of spinal anaesthesia
- Epidural anaesthesia is used to prevent autonomic hyperreflexia in parturients.

Reference

Hambly PR, Martin B. Anaesthesia for chronic spinal cord lesions. *Anaesthesia* March 1998, Volume 53(3), p273–289

Chronic obstructive pulmonary disease

A 64-year-old man presents to A+E extremely short of breath, initially unable to give a history. He is recognised by one of the nursing staff as a man known to have chronic obstructive pulmonary disease and was ventilated on ICU during his last admission.

How can we classify this disease?

There are some traditional definitions of chronic bronchitis and emphysema that have been linked clinically with the classical 'blue bloater' and 'pink puffer' respectively. There is, of course, a spectrum of disease and most patients will have elements of both.

- **Chronic bronchitis**   Defined as daily cough with sputum production for at least 3 months a year for at least 2 consecutive years

- **Emphysema**   A histological diagnosis defined as enlargement of the air spaces distal to the terminal bronchioles with destructive changes in the alveolar wall
- **'Blue bloater'**   This clinically represents the bronchitic group. They are typically hypoxaemic and cyanosed with cor pulmonale (peripheral oedema, raised JVP, hepatomegaly) but with little dyspnoea
- **'Pink puffers'**   Representing the emphysematous group. These patients have severe dyspnoea but relatively normal gas exchange

Can you tell me a little about the pathophysiology?

There is a combination of:

- Mucosal inflammation
- Excessive secretions
- Bronchoconstriction

There is a **reduction in lung elasticity** with consequent fall in the maximum expiratory flow rate. With increasing alveolar destruction the pulmonary vasculature may be damaged which, along with hypoxic pulmonary vasoconstriction, contributes to **pulmonary hypertension**. The overall effect is that of V/Q mismatch. Lung function tests show an obstructive picture:

- Reduced FEV_1
- Reduced FVC
- Reduced FEV_1/FVC ratio
- Increased residual volume
- Increased FRC
- Increased total lung capacity
- Reduced diffusing capacity

What signs might you elicit in this man?

- Tachypnoea
- Cyanosis
- Accessory muscle use
- Intercostal recession
- Hyperinflated lungs
- Pulsus paradoxus
- Wheeze
- Prolonged expiratory time
- Cor pulmonale   Raised JVP, peripheral oedema, loud P2
- Signs of hypercapnia   Warm peripheries, bounding pulse, confusion, tremor, convulsions

What would be your initial management of this man?

- ■ **Sit the patient up**
- ■ **Oxygen**   Initially in as high a concentration as possible to treat **life-threatening hypoxia** and then guided by blood gas analysis. The aim is to achieve a PaO_2 of at least 6.6 kPa without a fall in pH to below 7.26 (associated with poorer outcomes). **NB:** The BTS guidelines are as follows: 'In patients with a history of COPD aged 50 years or more, do not give an FiO_2 of more than 28% via a Venturi mask or 2 L/min via nasal cannulae until the arterial gas tensions are known.' This is contentious and is a view probably not shared by the majority of anaesthetists!
- ■ **Bronchodilators**   A proportion of these patients will have an element of reversibility to their bronchoconstriction. Use a β-agonist (salbutamol or terbutaline) with an anticholinergic (ipratropium bromide) Methylxanthines (aminophylline) can be used but there is little evidence to back up their effectiveness in this situation
- ■ **Steroids**   Still unclear if steroids alter **acute** exacerbations, but it is common practice to give 100 mg of hydrocortisone at presentation
- ■ **Antibiotics**   If clinically indicated
- ■ **Regular monitoring**   Clinical state and blood gases
- ■ **Heart failure Rx**   If indicated e.g. diuretics

BTS advocate the use of antibiotics if two or more of:

- ■ Increased breathlessness
- ■ Increased sputum volume
- ■ Development of purulent sputum

are present.

This man deteriorates despite all this treatment. What further interventions are available to you?

- ■ **Doxapram**   Sometimes considered to buy time
- ■ **Non-invasive ventilation**   Needs specialist equipment
  Needs co-operation from the patient
  Most valuable when used early
  Reduces requirement for IPPV and length of hospital stay
- ■ **IPPV**   Ventilatory support considered in patients:
  With a pH <7.26
  A rising $PaCO_2$
  Failing to respond to supportive treatment

Favourable factors for IPPV:

■ Remediable cause for acute decline
■ First episode
■ Good quality of life

Less favourable factors:

■ Documented severe COPD unresponsive to therapy
■ Poor quality of life, e.g. housebound on maximal therapy
■ Severe co-morbidities

References

Girou E *et al.* Association of noninvasive ventilation with nosocomial infection and survival in critically ill patients. *JAMA* Nov 8, 2000, Volume 284(18), p2361–2367

Management of acute exacerbations of COPD. *Thorax* 1997, Volume 52 (Suppl 5), S16–S21

Chronic renal failure

You are asked to anaesthetise a 40-year-old patient with chronic renal failure on haemodialysis for repair of a recurrent left inguinal hernia.

What anaesthetic problems do these patients present?

Renal patients have multiple medical problems that impact on anaesthesia. These include anaemia, coagulation disorders, cardiovascular pathology and disorders of other body systems. They also have altered drug handling.

Anaemia

Normochromic, normocytic (usually)

■ Multifactorial causes: Iron deficiency due to repeated blood loss with haemodialysis and associated peptic ulcer disease
B$_{12}$ and folate deficiency due to poor diet
Uraemia depresses erythropoietin production
Uraemia reduces red cell life span
■ Enquire about symptoms associated with anaemia, e.g. angina
■ Transfusion at Hb < 5 g/dl, or if symptoms are present, has been recommended
■ Low haemoglobins are tolerated because of the shift of the oxygen dissociation curve to the right ($\uparrow$ 2,3DPG and uraemic acidosis)
■ **NB:** Blood transfusion has effects on the immune system that may influence outcome after future transplantation

Blood clotting

▪ Patients with end-stage renal failure have abnormalities of platelet function due to defects in arachidonic acid metabolism and exposure of fibrinogen receptors
▪ Bleeding time is prolonged
▪ Risks and benefits of neuroaxial blocks need to be carefully assessed
▪ i.m. injections may be unwise

Cardiovascular system

▪ **Hypertension** Present in 80% of patients – usually on medication. Volatiles may exacerbate hypotensive effect. Exaggerated changes in BP and heart rate with induction and laryngoscopy
▪ **IHD**
▪ **CCF**
▪ Preoperative ECG, CXR and echocardiogram are necessary
▪ Carotid bruits – Doppler studies may be necessary
▪ Pericarditis – rare
▪ Endocarditis – especially if vascular access site is infected
▪ **Vascular access** – avoid forearm of non-dominant hand which should be preserved for a potential shunt
▪ AV fistulas should be kept warm and protected intraoperatively

Respiratory system

▪ SOB due to anaemia and acidosis
▪ Pulmonary oedema
▪ Pulmonary fibrosis associated with medical conditions
▪ Infection

Nervous system

▪ Neuropathy – autonomic (especially diabetics)/sensory/motor
▪ Myopathy due to uraemia causes an exaggerated response to muscle relaxants

Gastrointestinal system

▪ Delayed gastric emptying makes reflux and aspiration more likely
▪ **Rapid sequence induction** may be needed (?modified)
▪ Peptic ulceration
▪ Pre-medication should include an H_2 antagonist

Endocrine/Biochemical

▪ Hypocalcaemia and hypermagnesaemia (antacid consumption) potentiate relaxants
▪ Blood sugar should be monitored and controlled as many renal patients have diabetes
▪ Potassium rises in renal failure. Caution with suxamethonium and potassium-containing intravenous fluids (e.g. Hartmann's).

Renal system
- Ideal weight should be known
- A knowledge of daily urine volume normally passed and the dose of diuretic taken
- **CVP** monitoring may be needed to guide fluid management
- **Preoperative dialysis** and knowledge of potassium level post-dialysis
- **Intraoperative fluid**: avoid large volumes of crystalloid
- **Postoperative fluid**: previous hour's urine output plus insensible loss/h

How is drug handling altered in renal failure?

Many anaesthetic agents are potentiated in renal failure. This may be due to:

- Decreased protein binding
- Greater penetration of the blood–brain barrier
- Systemic effect of uraemia
- Elimination half-lives are prolonged

With respect to commonly used drugs:

- **Propofol** pharmacokinetics are unchanged
- **Thiopentone** and **benzodiazepines** can de reduced due to reduced protein binding
- **Morphine**, if used, must be carefully titrated as the metabolite morphine-6-glucuronide is active and accumulates
- **Atracurium** is the muscle relaxant of choice (Hofmann degradation)
- **NSAIDs** – avoid
- **Isoflurane** – safe
- **Enflurane** – avoid due to potential for nephrotoxicity from fluoride ions

---

Conduct of general anaesthesia:

Preop:	Medical assessment, dialysis, transfuse
	Premed – antacid
Intraop:	Monitoring – including CMV5, consider A-line and CVP
	Vascular access
	Induction – RSI
	Attention to pressor response
	Maintenance – IPPV, ↑FiO_2, N_2O safe
	Attention to fluid balance

Types of surgery common in renal patients:

- Vascular access procedures
- Peritoneal dialysis access
- Nephrectomy
- Renal transplant
- Parathyroidectomy

References

Holland DE, Old S. Anaesthesia for patients with impaired renal function. *Current Anaesthesia and Critical Care* 1992, Volume 3, p140–145

Morgan GE, Mikhail MS. *Clinical Anaesthesiology*, 2nd edition, 1996. Appleton and Lange, Stamford, CT

Complex regional pain syndrome

What do you understand by the term 'complex regional pain syndrome'?

There are two types of complex regional pain syndrome (CRPS) with defined diagnostic criteria:

- CRPS I   Formerly known as reflex sympathetic dystrophy or Sudeck's atrophy
- CRPS II   Formerly known as causalgia

Diagnostic criteria for CRPS I

1. An initiating noxious stimulus or cause of immobilisation.
2. Continuing symptoms (pain, allodynia, hyperalgesia) disproportionate to the initial event.
3. Evidence (at some time) of oedema, changes in skin blood flow or abnormal sudomotor (sweating) activity in the region of the pain.
4. Exclusion of other diagnoses.

Criteria 2,3 and 4 must be present.

Diagnostic criteria for CRPS II

1. Continuing pain, allodynia or hyperalgesia **following a nerve injury**, not necessarily limited to the distribution of the nerve.
2. Evidence (at some time) of oedema, changes in skin blood flow or abnormal sudomotor activity in the region of the pain
3. Exclusion of other diagnoses

Some chronic pain terminology:

Allodynia	Pain from a stimulus that does not normally cause pain
Hyperalgesia	A heightened response to a stimulus which is normally painful
Hyperpathia	Severe pain in an area of numbness

What are the clinical features?

■ Pain   A deep, burning pain localised to the limb
■ Allodynia
■ Hyperalgesia
■ Physical changes   Loss of hair
                              Trophic changes to the nails
                              Swelling and shininess
■ Temperature   The affected limb may be warm or cold
■ Localised osteoporosis   May or may not be present

> CRPS may be sympathetically maintained or sympathetically independent.

How might you manage this condition?

■ Restoration of mobility   Current management is based around gradually increasing function in the affected limb in conjunction with 'desensitisation', which exposes the limb to different sensory modalities. This is done by a multidisciplinary team in a quite specific way.
■ Determination of likely response to sympathetic blockade
■ If responsive, can try   Intravenous regional sympathetic blockade
                            Systemic sympathetic blockade
                            and physiotherapy
■ If unresponsive, can try   Antidepressants
                            Anticonvulsants
                            Capsaicin
                            and physiotherapy
■ Psychosocial support

Reference
Grady KM, Severn AM. *Key Topics in Chronic Pain*. Bios Scientific Publishers, 1997, Oxford

Diabetes: Perioperative management

An elderly patient with IDDM is scheduled for an axillo-femoral bypass graft.

What are the important features of a preoperative assessment in diabetic patients?

Glycaemic control
It is important to get a feel for the patient's recent diabetic control, assessing glucose control as well as hydration and acid–base balance. Current hypoglycaemic agents should be reviewed. The patient will undergo a period of starvation as well as a surge of catabolic hormone secretion associated with the stress response to surgery.

Tight control of blood glucose has both short- and long-term advantages. In the **acute setting** inadequately treated diabetes can cause symptomatic hypoglycaemic episodes or severe dehydration with acidosis (lactic and/or ketoacids). Raised blood sugar levels perioperatively have been linked with wound infection and poor neurological outcome in cardiac surgery.

In the **longer term**, improved glucose control can reduce the microvascular and neuropathic complications of this disease.

Assessment of diabetic complications
- Coronary artery disease
- Autonomic neuropathy
- Diabetic nephropathy
- Respiratory changes/airway assessment
- Associated endocrine disorders

Are these complications of diabetes of concern to you as an anaesthetist?

- Diabetics are 4–5 times as likely to have coronary heart disease as non-diabetics and a proportion of these are asymptomatic.
- **Autonomic neuropathy** occurs in up to 40% of type 1 diabetics and can take the form of postural hypotension, gastroparesis, diarrhoea and bladder paresis. There can be **unexpected tachycardia, arrhythmias and hypotension** (often unresponsive to atropine and ephedrine). Diabetics with autonomic neuropathy show **increased QT variability** (i.e. regional variations in ventricular recovery) and this may be a major factor in the 'sudden death syndrome' recognised in this group. **Gastroparesis** causes an increase in the volume of gastric contents with increased risk of aspiration. The degree of autonomic neuropathy is difficult to quantify preoperatively but the Valsalva manoeuvre and assessment of heart rate variability may be of benefit.
- **Diabetic nephropathy** increases the risk of perioperative renal failure and infection. Appropriate fluid and haemodynamic monitoring is essential.
- **Respiratory**: diabetes is associated with a reduced FEV_1 and FVC. It has been estimated that 30–40% of long-standing diabetics develop the **'stiff joint**

syndrome' in which chronically raised blood sugar levels cause protein glycosylation and reduced elasticity of connective tissues. This is associated with poor neck extension and mouth opening and a higher incidence of difficult intubation.

How would you manage this man's glucose control perioperatively?

This is an elderly man who is insulin dependent undergoing a major surgical procedure. The main principles are:

■ Regular blood glucose monitoring
■ Insulin and glucose infusions during the period of starvation

There are many methods of providing continuous insulin/glucose infusions and hospital policy may dictate the regimen chosen. The two main regimens are:

1. Separate infusions of insulin and glucose – the insulin rate is adjusted according to the blood glucose level
2. The Alberti regimen provides glucose, insulin and potassium in the same solution, thus eliminating the potential for giving insulin without glucose or vice versa

As indicated above, these regimens should be commenced and stabilised preoperatively and continued until the patient has resumed eating/drinking and their normal hypoglycaemic agents.

What is your preferred anaesthetic technique in this man?

This man requires a general anaesthetic and if gastric stasis is suspected then a rapid sequence induction is the technique of choice. In an elderly man with known vascular disease, an arterial line inserted pre-induction would be prudent especially if there is a question of autonomic neuropathy. A high-dose opiate anaesthetic technique will reduce the sympathetic and hormonal response to surgery, providing both metabolic and haemodynamic stability.

Reference
McAnulty GR, Robertshaw HJ, Hall GM. Anaesthetic management of patients with diabetes mellitus. *BJA*, July 2000, Volume 85(1), p80–90

Diabetic ketoacidosis

What is the mechanism of ketone production in diabetes?

Ketones are **produced from acetyl-CoA in the liver mitochondria** and are used as fuel by the brain and muscle. Acetyl-CoA is the end product of β-**oxidation** of fatty acids. If there is **excess fatty acid breakdown** (as in diabetes and starvation) then there will not be enough oxaloacetate to join with all the acetyl-CoA in order for it to enter the citric acid cycle. In this situation the

excess acetyl-CoA is diverted into ketone production. The accumulation of ketoacids (β-**hydroxybutyrate and aceto-acetate**) cause a metabolic acidosis when levels reach about 10 mmol/L. The rate of production is usually slow but can be as fast as 1 mmol/min.

Conditions required for ketone production

- **Insulin deficiency.** However, only a very low level of insulin is required to inhibit hepatic ketogenesis
- **Counter-regulatory hormone excess** (an increase in glucagon, catecholamines and glucocorticoids)

> **Further pathophysiology . . .**
>
> Insulin lack accelerates glycogenolysis and gluconeogenesis. An **osmotic diuresis** results from the high blood glucose and causes uncontrolled urinary loss of K^+, Na^+ and water. This **decreased ECF volume** leads to pre-renal failure. Renal excretion of glucose is then inhibited which leads to a further increase in plasma glucose level. Hyperglycaemia moves water out of cells into the ECF. This can decrease the serum $[Na^+]$. Nausea and vomiting frequently complicate the biochemical picture.

What are the actions of insulin?

Insulin prevents proteolysis, glycogenolysis and lipolysis and promotes uptake and storage of fuel. It is an anabolic hormone. Insulin binds to a specific membrane-bound receptor and alters intracellular cAMP levels.

Carbohydrate
- **Increases glycogen synthesis** (phosphofructokinase and glycogen synthase)
- **Inhibits glycogenolysis and gluconeogenesis**
- **The increased uptake of glucose** into cells (such as adipose tissue and muscles) by increased glucokinase activity is now considered much less important

Fat
- **Decreases triglyceride breakdown** in adipocytes (triglyceride-lipase)
- **Increases fatty acid synthesis** in the liver due to activation of acetyl CoA carboxylase
- **Activates lipoprotein lipase**, which splits triglycerides enabling the fatty acids to enter adipose tissue for storage
- **Increases esterification** of fatty acids with glycerol in adipose tissue

Protein
- **Decreases proteolysis**
- **Increases uptake of amino acids** into cells
- **Increases mRNA translation**

Increased K^+ and Mg^{2+} transport into cells.

How would you manage a diabetic with ketoacidosis?

Treatment of DKA needs to address:

■ **Fluid deficit/Shock**
■ **Insulin deficiency**
■ **Hypokalaemia**
■ **Acidosis**
■ **Underlying/precipitating cause**

History

Examination
■ Sunken eyes
■ Reduced skin turgor
■ Acetone smell on breath
■ Kussmaul's breathing
■ Low BP
■ Decreased conscious level

Investigations
■ **Arterial blood gases** for acid–base balance
■ **Anion gap**
■ **Plasma glucose**
■ **Plasma Na$^+$ concentration** is usually low as an osmolar compensation for the high glucose. If the sodium is high this represents severe water loss
■ **Plasma K$^+$ concentration** may be high on presentation, but the total body potassium is low due to the absence of insulin allowing it to drift out of the cells.
■ **Urea and creatinine**   Pre-renal failure from ECF depletion
                             Diabetic nephropathy
■ **Osmolality** of serum
■ **Serum/Urinary ketones** (aceto-acetate). The ratio of β-hydroxybutyrate to aceto-acetate is governed by pH. As the pH decreases the ratio increases. Conventional bedside tests for ketones only react with acetoacetic acid and therefore it is possible to have a very high β-hydroxybutyrate concentration and have the test only show a trace of ketones
■ **PO$_4$** levels tend to follow K$^+$
■ **CXR, ECG, FBC, blood cultures, urine culture and sputum culture** to look for underlying cause

Monitoring
■ ECG/Heart rate/BP/Temp./Resp. rate/Urine output/NG tube
■ Regular blood glucose monitoring
■ HDU/ICU

Treatment

■ **ECF volume** should be replaced with **normal saline** (CVP line may be needed)
  Start with 1–2 litres in the first hour. More than 6 litres may be needed
■ **Insulin** (actrapid) at 0.1 unit/kg bolus and then 0.1 unit/kg/hour
■ **Potassium** replacement should begin when serum [K+] becomes less than 4.5 mmol/L. 20 mmol/hour if K+ is 4–5 mmol/L, 40 mmol/hour if 3–4 and 40–60 mmol/hour if <3 mmol/L
■ **5% or 10% Dextrose** should be started when the plasma glucose falls below 14 mmol/L
■ **Bicarbonate therapy** is controversial. Several centres use it if pH < 7.0 or if the [HCO_3^-] is <5.0 mmol/L
  The problems with it are: Large Na^+ load
                              Increased CO_2 production (may easily enter cells and cause a paradoxical intracellular acidosis)
                              Hypokalaemia
                              Metabolic alkalosis as ketoacids disappear
                              Left-shift of oxyhaemoglobin dissociation curve
■ **Phosphate therapy** has no proven benefit
■ **The underlying cause** must be treated (myocardial infarction, infection, etc.)

Anion gap

$$= (Na^+ + K^+) - (HCO_3^- + Cl^-)$$

■ Normal value = 10–18 mmol/L
■ Represents unmeasured anions, e.g. albumin, sulphate and phosphate
■ An increase is due to an unmeasured anion that is balanced by H^+ causing an acidosis e.g. lactate or ketoacids

---

Complications

■ Shock and lactic acidosis
■ Coma
■ Cerebral oedema
■ Hypothermia
■ DVT
■ Iatrogenic electrolyte imbalance

References

Goguen JM, Josse RG. Management of diabetic ketoacidosis. *Medicine International,* July 1993, Volume 21(7), p275–278
Kumar PJ, Clark ML. *Clinical Medicine,* 3rd edition, 1994. Baillière Tindall, London
Sonksen P, Sonksen J. Insulin: understanding its action in health and disease. *BJA,* July 2000, Volume 85 (1), p69–79
The Oxford Textbook of Medicine, 3rd edition, 1996. Oxford University Press.
Viallon A *et al.* Does bicarbonate therapy improve the management of severe diabetic ketoacidosis? *Critical Care Medicine,* Dec 1999, Volume 27(12), p2690–2693

Down's syndrome

A 7-year-old boy with Down's syndrome is scheduled to undergo a 90 minute dental conservation procedure.

What is Down's syndrome?

Down's syndrome (Trisomy 21) occurs in approximately 1:600 births (the commonest congenital abnormality). The incidence increases with increasing maternal age and the majority (> 90%) have an extra chromosome 21 because of non-dysjunction at the time of gamete formation. It less commonly results from translocation and it is these parents that are at great risk of having further affected children.

What are the features of Down's syndrome?

No single feature is pathognomonic of the syndrome but the association of several signs can usually lead to a clinical diagnosis. These include:

■ Skull	Flattened face and occiput
	3rd fontanelle
■ Eyes	Prominent epicanthic folds
	Oblique palpebral fissure
	Brushfield spots
	Squint, nystagmus
	Cataracts
■ Digits	Single palmar (Simian) crease
	Short fingers
	Wide gap between 1st and 2nd toes
■ Respiratory	Macroglossia (50%)
	Micrognathia
	High arched palate (70%)
	Subglottic stenosis
	Upper airway obstruction (tonsillar/adenoidal hypertrophy)
	Increased susceptibility to respiratory infections
	Atlantoaxial instability (15%)
	Short, broad neck
■ Heart	40% have some sort of cardiac abnormality
■ CNS	Developmental delay
	Epilepsy
■ Endocrine	Hypothyroidism (40%)
■ Immune	Leukaemia (risk increased by 20 times)
	Immunosuppression

Cardiac abnormalities associated with Down's syndrome:

■ Endocardial cushion defects	40%
■ VSD	27%
■ PDA	12%
■ Fallot's tetralogy	8%
■ Others	13%

What abnormalities are relevant to anaesthesia?

Airway management

Patients with Down's syndrome have a large, protruding tongue, a small mandible and an increased incidence of subglottic stenosis leading to difficult intubation and the need for a smaller tracheal tube than expected.

Atlantoaxial instability occurs in about 15% and is due to laxity of the transverse atlantal ligament. It is asymptomatic in most cases, particularly if the atlantoaxial distance is less than 6 mm. Care must be taken when manipulating the head and neck during laryngoscopy/intubation and during anaesthesia in general because of reduced muscle tone. There is still debate as to whether all Down's patients should have cervical spine X-rays prior to anaesthesia. The current consensus seems to be that those who are symptomatic should be X-rayed.

Careful assessment of the airway and review of previous anaesthesia records may give some indication as to the expected ease of laryngoscopy.

Post-extubation stridor, postoperative chest infections and pulmonary oedema are more common than in the normal population.

Cardiac

The cardiac abnormalities associated with Down's syndrome are outlined above. The main clinical problem is pulmonary hypertension which may also be present in the absence of an anatomical lesion (? related to chronic anaemia). Anaesthesia is based around controlling the balance between pulmonary and systemic vascular resistance.

Prophylactic antibiotics may be necessary.

Mental retardation

May cause difficulties with cooperation at induction.

Associated epilepsy

Higher incidence of hepatitis B in institutionalised patients

Reference

Mitchell V, Howard R, Facer E. Down's syndrome and anaesthesia. *Paediatric Anaesthesia,* 1995, Volume 5, p379–384

Dural Tap ✓

You are performing an epidural on a 23-year-old primigravida in labour. As you advance your Tuohy needle, you notice clear fluid coming out.

What are you going to do?

There are two alternative strategies in this situation:

- **Resite the epidural** – the commonest approach involves resiting the epidural in an adjacent space. The obvious anxiety is that some of the solution may subsequently pass into the subarachnoid space. To avoid a high block, the local anaesthetic doses should be given in smaller and divided doses (and by an anaesthetist). Post-delivery, an infusion of crystalloid may be continued epidurally to try and reduce the incidence of headache.
- **Use a subarachnoid catheter** – some anaesthetists will insert an end-hole catheter and give increments of local anaesthetic (0.5–1 ml of 0.5% heavy or plain bupivacaine) to achieve analgesia. CSF catheters may reduce the incidence of headache by causing a fibroblast reaction and sealing the tear.

What will you tell the obstetricians?

Traditionally, there was a view that these women should not be allowed to have an active second stage and were often delivered with forceps. This, however, does not seem to reduce the incidence of post-dural puncture headache and current practice allows **normal delivery providing the second stage is not prolonged**. For this reason, the obstetrician should be informed.

Tell me about the pathophysiology of post-dural puncture headache.

Inadvertent spinal tap is a well-recognised complication of epidural analgesia and the incidence is around 1% in obstetric practice. Headache occurs in around 80%, typically from 2–24 hours postpuncture. The headache is thought to be due to **loss of CSF via the tear resulting in traction on the intracranial contents**. A reduction in CSF pressure may lead to cerebral vasodilatation and headache and some therapies e.g. sumatriptan assume this to be part of the problem.

What are the signs and symptoms of post-dural puncture headache?

- Severe postural headache with a temporal relationship to a dural puncture
- Typically bilateral and occipital/frontal
- Neck ache
- Nausea and vomiting
- Photophobia
- Rarely there can be cranial nerve palsies

It is usually self-limiting but can last for months and is associated with significant morbidity.

What would your initial management be?

- Full explanation to the mother
- Bed rest (as far as is practical)
- Adequate hydration
- Simple analgesics
- Stool softeners

- Epidural saline could be considered
- Others – i.v. caffeine, sumatriptan

When and how would you perform an epidural blood patch?

- **When**   **After 24 h**
              It has been demonstrated (Loeser *et al* 1978) that a patch
              performed within 24 hours has a 70% failure rate while a patch
              after 24 hours has a failure rate of 4%. The initial 24 hours is
              generally managed conservatively and if the headache persists,
              blood patching is discussed with the patient. Magnetic resonance
              imaging (Beards *et al* 1993) has shown that the dural tear is
              indeed patched by the injected blood and together with a mass
              effect acts to increase CSF pressure. A single blood patch leads to
              resolution of symptoms in 80–90% of patients with a success rate
              of 95% after a second patch.

- **How**   Two anaesthetists (one a consultant)
              Aseptic technique performed in theatre
              Locate epidural space at or just below site of dural tap
              20 ml of patient's blood taken aseptically
              Slow injection of blood into epidural space
              Stop injecting if pain or paraesthesia (otherwise 20 ml injected)
              Place patient supine

References
Beards SC *et al*. Magnetic resonance imaging of extradural blood patches: appearances from
      30 min to 18 h. *BJA*, August 1993, Volume 71(2), p182–188
Loeser EA *et al*. Time versus success rate for epidural blood patch. *Anesthesiology*, August 1978,
      Volume 49, p147–149

Eisenmenger's syndrome

You are asked to anaesthetise a 16-year-old male patient who has Down's syndrome and Eisenmenger's syndrome. The patient has a mental age of 6 years. He presents for emergency surgery with a cold, white, pulseless and painful left leg. This is obviously a complicated case!

What is Eisenmenger's syndrome?

This exists in any condition in which communication between the systemic and pulmonary circulations gives rise to pulmonary hypertension ultimately resulting in right-to-left shunt. This functional reversal causes cyanosis.

Eisenmenger's syndrome may be associated with:

- ASD
- VSD
- PDA
- Other complex anomalies

What are the general principles of anaesthetising this patient?

When anaesthetising this patient there will be problems related to:
- Down's syndrome (see question on Down's syndrome)
- Eisenmenger's syndrome
- Emergency anaesthesia

What are the principles of anaesthetising a patient with Eisenmenger's syndrome?

The key points are:

- **Managing the balance between SVR and PVR.** A drop in SVR (or a rise in PVR) will increase the right-to-left shunt. PVR is fairly fixed in these patients and therefore difficult to manipulate. Factors that increase PVR are:
  Hypoxia
  Hypercarbia
  N_2O
  Histamine, serotonin, noradrenaline
  Low lung volumes

Under anaesthesia, the **SVR is far more prone to change**. Most induction agents decrease SVR and therefore would result in an increase in cyanosis.

Ketamine has been used for induction (although it increases PVR as well). Noradrenaline and metaraminol have been used to maintain SVR. Atropine may be needed to prevent reflex bradycardia.

- **SBE prophylaxis**
- **Care with i.v. injections to avoid paradoxical air embolus**
- **Maintenance of adequate circulating volume**
- **Avoid myocardial depressants**

How is the speed of both gas and intravenous induction affected by the presence of a right-to-left shunt?

■ **Gas induction** This is slower because the blood from the lungs (which has equilibrated with alveolar anaesthetic gases) is 'diluted' by the blood, with a low partial pressure, which has bypassed the lungs. The resulting brain partial pressure of agent is therefore slower to equilibrate with alveolar gas.
■ **Intravenous induction** This is quicker because some of the agent will behave like a 'paradoxical embolus' and enter the systemic circulation, bypassing the lungs, causing a rapid rise in brain concentration.

What may be the cause of the ischaemic leg?

It may be due to a paradoxical embolus, for example from a deep vein thrombosis passing through the defect in the heart. It could also be thrombus from the atria if the patient is in atrial fibrillation.

Eisenmenger's Complex:	Original description in 1897 at post-mortem Pulmonary vascular disease in the presence of VSD and right ventricular hypertrophy
Eisenmenger's syndrome:	Redefined in 1958 by Wood Pulmonary hypertension at the systemic level caused by high pulmonary vascular resistance with reversed or bidirectional shunt via a large VSD.

Although both definitions refer to a VSD, the site of the communication is not important.

References

Bird TM, Strunin L. Anaesthesia for a patient with Down's syndrome and Eisenmenger's complex. *Anaesthesia* 1984, Volume 39, p48–50

Goldstone JC, Pollard BJ. *Adult congenital heart disease: specific examples. Handbook of Clinical Anaesthesia*, 1996. Churchill Livingstone, Edinburgh

Mather SJ, Hughes DG. *A Handbook of Paediatric Anaesthesia*, 2nd edition, 1996. Oxford Medical Publications, Oxford

Sammut MS, Paes ML. Anaesthesia for laparoscopic cholecystectomy in a patient with Eisenmenger's syndrome. *BJA* 1997, Volume 79, p810–812

Guillain–Barré syndrome

You are called to see a 25-year-old man on a medical ward with a 10-day history of progressive weakness.

What is the differential diagnosis?

- Guillain–Barré syndrome
- Motor neurone disease
- Multiple sclerosis
- Polyneuropathy – polio, HIV
- Hypo/hyperkalaemic periodic paralysis (or iatrogenic)

What is the clinical picture of Guillain–Barré syndrome?

This syndrome is characterised by:

- **Progressive, symmetrical, ascending flaccid motor weakness**
- Around 80% have **sensory symptoms** (pain is very common)
- Around 65% have **autonomic dysfunction**
- It is often preceded by an infective illness

The age-specific curve shows a bimodal distribution with peaks in young adults and the elderly. Males are more commonly affected. The main problems in the acute situation are:

- **Respiratory failure** requiring assisted ventilation due to progression of the paralysis to involve respiratory muscles
- **Autonomic neuropathy** which can be severe causing orthostatic hypotension and cardiac arrhythmias

> Disease named after two case reports by Guillain, Barré and Strohl in 1916.
> The full spectrum of GBS ranges from acute inflammatory demyelinating polyneuropathy to the pure motor variants and the Miller–Fisher syndrome.
> Miller–Fisher syndrome (1956) describes the association of ophthalmoplegia, ataxia and areflexia.

What are the causes of this syndrome?

The syndrome may be an immune reaction triggered by either infection or vaccination.
   Antecedent *infections* include:

- **Campylobacter** — *Campylobacter jejuni*, a major cause of bacterial gastroenteritis worldwide, is the most frequent antecedent pathogen (up to 45% in some studies)
- **Cytomegalovirus** — The second commonest associated infection which particularly affects young females

- **Epstein–Barr virus**
- **Mycoplasma**
- **Association with HIV**

It is likely that immune responses directed towards the infecting organisms are involved in the pathogenesis by cross-reaction with neural tissues.

Possible associated *vaccinations* include influenza, polio, rabies and rubella. Most large-scale epidemiological studies have failed to find a cause–effect relationship. In up to 30% of cases no cause is found.

There is **widespread segmental demyelination of peripheral nerves**. Cerebrospinal fluid typically shows few cells with a high protein content (in 90% of cases), though the diagnosis remains a clinical one.

Why or when might you intubate these patients?

Around 25% of patients require mechanical ventilation, so close monitoring must be ensured should a deterioration in respiratory function occur. Forced vital capacity (FVC) should be measured regularly. There are no 'rules' regarding mechanical ventilation. However:

- Some recommend ventilation if the FVC < 1L (others < 10–15 ml/kg)
- The speed of deterioration will also influence any decisions
- Other factors, e.g. aspiration, bulbar weakness should be taken into account

Early tracheostomy is recommended.

Do you know of any specific treatments?

Plasma exchange	Involves the removal of about 200 ml/kg of plasma over 4–6 sessions and replacement with colloid or crystalloid Thought to work by removal of a humoral demyelinating factor. This treatment does not influence mortality but reduces the ventilation and complication rate
Immunoglobulin	Intravenously for 5 days Much more convenient than plasma exchange Randomised control trials show that immuno-globulin and plasma exchange are equally effective in reducing the time to functional recovery
Immunosuppressants	Steroids and other immunosuppressants are no longer recommended

What other problems might they encounter on ICU?

- Pneumonia
- Line infections
- DVT

- ■ Nutritional deficits
- ■ Psychological — There should be early and active psychological support for the patient and relatives
- ■ Autonomic neuropathy — Ensure adequate circulating volume and sedation β-blockers; atropine and pacemakers have all been used to manage autonomic disturbances
- ■ Pain — Pain is common (especially in the back and lower limbs) and can be a major problem. Opiates are often required. A randomised, double-blind crossover trial showed that carbamazepine is a useful adjuvant for pain control, reducing narcotic requirements. Intensive physiotherapy is essential
- ■ GI haemorrhage

Do you know the prognosis?

Around 80% make a near complete recovery although the speed of recovery is variable. At least 10% will have a significant permanent disability and the mortality rate is 5–10%.

Poorer prognosis is associated with:

- ■ Older patients
- ■ Preceding *Campylobacter jejuni* infection
- ■ Need for mechanical ventilation
- ■ Rapid progression of symptoms
- ■ Extensive disease

References

Hinds CJ, Watson D. *Neurological disorders, Intensive Care, A Concise Textbook*. 2nd edition, 1996. Baillière Tindall, London

Seneviratne U. Guillain–Barré syndrome. *Postgrad Med J*, 2000, Volume 76, p774–782

Tripathi M, Kaushik S. Carbamazepine for pain management in Guillain–Barré syndrome patients in the intensive care unit. *Crit Care Med*, March 2000, Volume 28(3), p655–658

Heart block and temporary pacing

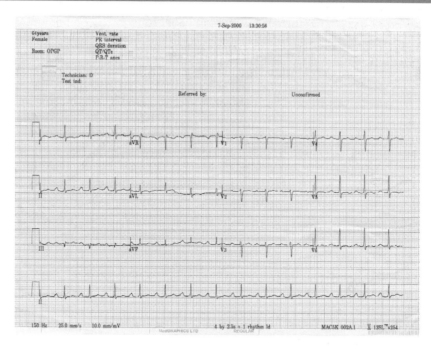

Have a look at this ECG. What does it show?

The ECG shows sinus rhythm at a rate of 87 beats per minute. The axis is normal. The PR interval is prolonged. There are no other abnormalities. The diagnosis is first degree heart block.

How do you know it is first-degree heart block?

The normal PR interval is 120–210 milliseconds (some books say 200 ms!). The PR interval is measured from the start of the P wave to the start of the ventricular complex, whether that is a Q or an R wave. At a standard paper speed of 25 mm/s, each small square is equivalent to 40 ms. The normal PR interval is therefore 3–5(ish) small squares.

What types of heart block are there?

The term 'heart block' usually refers to atrio-ventricular block as distinct from 'bundle-branch' block.

Atrio-ventricular heart block is classified into first-, second- or third-degree depending on the effect on atrio-ventricular conduction.

- **First-degree**   As described above.
- **Second-degree**   Mobitz type I (or Wenkebach)
  Mobitz type II
  In **Mobitz type I** block the PR interval increases successively with each beat until a QRS complex is

'dropped'. When seen in young, fit people (often nocturnally) with high vagal tone it may be benign. When it cannot be attributed to high vagal tone it may have a similar prognosis to Mobitz type II

In **Mobitz type II** block there is intermittent failure of A–V conduction. This results in 2:1 or 3:1 A–V block, for example. The block is usually below the A–V node and is associated with an increased incidence of Stokes–Adams attacks, slow ventricular rates and sudden death.

■ **Third-degree**   There is total interruption of A–V conduction such that the ventricular 'escape' rate bears no relation to the atrial rate. The ventricular rate is determined by the site of the block, which may be nodal or infra-nodal. A nodal block resulting in a His-bundle pacemaker may have a fairly 'normal' rate and narrow QRS complexes. An infra-nodal block resulting in a pacemaker from the left or right bundle-branch will have a slow rate with broad QRS complexes.

What are the indications for pacing pre-operatively?

Suggested indications include:

■ Acute anterior myocardial infarction (MI)
■ Acute MI with Mobitz type II or third-degree block (?also new BBB)
■ First-degree heart block with bifascicular block
■ Any symptomatic bradyarrhythmia
■ Refractory supra-ventricular tachyarrhythmia

How may peri-operative pacing be achieved?

■ **Transthoracic non-invasive**   The anterior patch must be negative and placed just to the left of the xiphoid process to avoid the pectoral muscle-mass. The posterior patch is placed inferior to the left scapula

■ **Epicardial**   Usually performed by surgeons during cardiac surgery

■ **Transvenous**   May or may not be balloon-tipped to help with insertion. Requires X-ray control to check its position in the apex of the right ventricle (pointing down). A pacing wire that is pointing towards the left shoulder may be in the coronary sinus

■ **Transoesophageal**   Used when slow atrial rhythm. Left atrium lies anterior to the oesophagus. The pacer is switched on and advanced until capture occurs (usually at 30–35 cm from teeth)

References

Bennett DH. *Cardiac Arrhythmias*, 4th edition, 1994. BH publishing, Oxford

Bourke M.E. The patient with a pacemaker or related device. *Canadian Journal of Anaesthesia* 1996, Volume 43, No.5 (part 2), R24–32

Deakin CD. *Clinical Notes for the FRCA*, 1998. Churchill Livingstone, Edinburgh

Morgan GE, Mikhail MS. *Clinical Anaesthesiology*, 2nd edition, 1996. Appleton and Lange, Stamford, CT

ICU neuropathy

What are the causes of muscle weakness in critically ill patients?

> This could bring up an enormous list of the various causes and it helps to
> think for a few moments to try and categorise the main areas for
> discussion. The examiners will use this opening question to close down in
> more detail on one of two subjects they wish to discuss.

A suitable classification might be:

■ **Pre-existing medical conditions**
Guillain–Barré syndrome
Myasthenia gravis
CNS lesions e.g. trauma, polio, MND
■ **Drug related** Muscle relaxants
Aminoglycosides (may interfere with
neuromuscular transmission)
Magnesium (in pre-eclampsia)
Steroids (typically proximal weakness/wasting)
Poisoning, e.g. botulinum toxin, organophosphates
■ **Metabolic** Hypokalaemia
Hypophosphataemia
■ **Myopathy** (acquired) Immobilization, disuse atrophy
Malnutrition, leading to muscle wasting and
weakness. A paper in the *BMJ* in 1994 showed that
up to 40% of patients (not ICU) are undernourished
at presentation and that there is an average loss of
5.4% body weight in hospital. Therefore, ICU
patients are often malnourished and catabolic.
Protein turnover is increased secondary to surgery,
trauma and critical illness.
Critical illness myopathy
■ **Critical illness neuropathy**

Tell me a bit more about critical illness neuropathy.

This is an acquired neuropathy commonly found in association with severe
sepsis and multiple organ failure (50–70% of these patients). It has been
recognised as a clinical entity since 1983 when described by Bolton *et al*. The
cause remains unknown and there is no specific treatment. It can often come
to light in recovering patients who are slow or difficult to wean from
mechanical ventilation.

Neurophysiological studies show relatively **preserved nerve conduction
velocities with primary axonal degeneration of motor and sensory nerves.**
Clinically there is a flaccid weakness with absent/reduced tendon reflexes and
muscle wasting. CSF protein levels are normal (c.f. Guillain–Barré) and CK

levels are normal or slightly elevated. Recovery from the neuropathy generally lags behind resolution of the underlying ICU diagnosis and physiotherapy is needed during rehabilitation. In those who survive the underlying MODS, the prognosis is good with full or near full recovery the most common outcome.

References
Bolton C et al. The electrophysiological investigation of respiratory paralysis in critically ill patients. Neurology 1983, Volume 33(suppl), p186

Gutmann MD. Critical illness neuropathy and myopathy. Arch Neurol. May 1999, p527–528

McWhirter JP, Pennington CR. Incidence and recognition of malnutrition in hospital. BMJ 1994, Volume 308, p945–948

ICU nutrition

Why is nutritional support important in ICU patients?

A significant number of patients admitted to hospital are malnourished, up to 40% according to McWhirter. The majority of patients that are admitted to intensive care are catabolic and will have had a preceding period of starvation due to their surgery or underlying pathology.

Complications of poor nutritional support

- Impaired wound healing
- Reduced muscle bulk/strength and delayed mobilisation
- Increased incidence of respiratory infection
- Problems with weaning from mechanical ventilation

How can you make an assessment of a patient's nutritional status on ICU?

There are **objective markers** that can be used in the assessment of *malnutrition* but many of these are flawed when faced with a patient with multiorgan failure on intensive care. There are other methods that are more clinically orientated.

Traditional objective assessment tools
- Triceps skinfold thickness
- Hand grip tests
- Serum albumin ($t_{1/2}$ 14–20 days)
- Serum prealbumin ($t_{1/2}$ 24–48 hours)
- Serum transferrin
- Total iron-binding capacity
- Lymphocyte count

These are relatively insensitive and non-specific markers e.g. serum albumin is affected by trauma, sepsis and excess extracellular water.

Other methods

■ Subjective global assessment (SGA) – history and physical factors
■ Hill and Windsor (bedside nutritional assessment)

Lean body mass assessment – experimental methods

■ Bioimpedence
■ Measuring total body water or potassium
■ Neutron activation
■ Muscle biopsy to measure muscle fibre area

These methods are similarly difficult to interpret in a critical care setting.
   A nutritional history should be elicited (including normal weight and recent food intake) and there are formulae to derive ideal body mass and daily calorific requirements.

> This question initially seems difficult to answer (as rarely formally done on ICU).
> Your answer should emphasise that a detailed history and examination are still the mainstay of nutritional assessment.
> However, you will need to be aware of the tests available.
> Be wary of starting your answer with a negative comment about how difficult it is to assess nutritional status on ICU – perhaps mention this at the end, with the reasons why.

What routes can be used for nutritional support?

Nutrition can be provided either by:

■ **Enteral feeding**	Can be given by **nasogastric, nasojejunal or percutaneous gastrostomy/jejunostomy** tubes. Post-pyloric feeding is becoming more popular as gastric atony can be a problem in critically ill patients
■ **Parenteral feeding**	Often through a dedicated central venous catheter, although peripheral polyurethane catheters or peripherally inserted central catheters (PICC) can be used

What problems are associated with parenteral nutrition?

■ Central venous catheter	Complications related to insertion
	Catheter-related sepsis
	Displacement
	Occlusion/thrombosis
■ Metabolic	Hypo/**hyper**glycaemia
	Metabolic acidosis
	Potassium, sodium and phosphate imbalance

	Excess CO_2 production
	Hypercholesterolaemia/hypertriglyceridaemia
	Essential fatty acid/vitamins/trace element deficiencies
▧ Intestinal	TPN fails to reverse intestinal villous atrophy and bacterial translocation can occur
▧ Hepatobiliary	Abnormal liver function tests. This is multifactorial
▧ Refeeding syndrome	↓ Glu, $MgSO_4$, K^+, PO_4 seen when refeeding malnourished patients

What are the advantages of enteral nutrition?

- ▧ More physiological route for digestion and absorption
- ▧ Prevents mucosal atrophy – intestinal enterocytes receive a proportion of their own nutrition directly from the gut lumen and enteral nutrition helps maintain mucosal blood flow
- ▧ Supports the normal gut flora
- ▧ Reduction of bacterial translocation – ↓ **risk of sepsis**
- ▧ Fewer metabolic complications
- ▧ No catheter-associated complications of TPN – in particular the risk of central line sepsis

What can you tell me about immunomodulation and feeding?

Critically ill patients have impaired gastrointestinal function (motility, secretions, mucosal atrophy, altered flora and bacterial translocation) secondary to an acute phase response. Increased bacterial translocation is associated with an increased risk of sepsis. To reduce this, there has been interest in dietary components with immunomodulatory properties.

▧ **Glutamine**	The most abundant amino acid in the body
	Fuel for enterocytes and some lymphoid cells
	Becomes a *conditionally* essential amino acid in critical illness
	Can significantly reduce mortality and length of stay
▧ **Arginine**	Promotes T-cell proliferation, macrophage and natural killer cell function
	Role in nitric oxide formation
▧ **Taurine**	Becomes a *conditionally* essential amino acid in critical illness
	Antioxidant
	Modulates inflammatory cytokines
▧ **Omega-3 fatty acids**	Anti-inflammatory activity via prostaglandin
▧ **Ribonucleotides**	Promote protein synthesis

> **Typical daily nutritional requirements:**
> Water   30 ml/kg
> Na+   1.2 mmol/kg
> K+   0.8 mmol/kg
> Calories   30 kcal/kg
> Protein   0.3 g nitrogen
> Fat   2 g/kg
> Glucose   2 g/kg

References

Edmonson WC. Nutritional support in critical care. *BJA*, Feb 2001. CEPD reviews, Volume 1, No.1
Lalwani K. Current aspects of parenteral nutrition. *Anaesthesia Review*, 1997, Volume 13, p201–221.
    Churchill Livingstone

ICU stress ulceration

Can you tell me something about the pathophysiology of stress ulcers in intensive care patients?

Stress ulceration in intensive care patients is relatively common (approaching 90% by day 3 with no prophylaxis), although the incidence of clinically important gastrointestinal bleeding is less than 2%. However, the risk is significantly increased in two subgroups of patients:

■ Respiratory failure requiring mechanical ventilation for more than 48 h
■ Coagulopathy

The normal mechanisms that aim to ensure an intact mucosal barrier to protect the gastric epithelium come under attack in the critically ill patient.

■ Mucus production is reduced from surface mucous cells
■ Mucosal blood flow is impaired
■ Mucosal prostaglandin production is reduced and these (especially PGE2) are involved in the regulation of gastric acid secretion by parietal cells. Prostaglandins normally inhibit acid secretion by activating Gi, thereby reducing adenylyl cyclase activity and cAMP production. CyclicAMP in turn regulates H^+ transport via protein kinases and $H^+K^+ATPase$
■ Other factors may include increased gastrin production, acid–base abnormalities and reflux of bile

The result is an imbalance between acid secretion and normal protective mucus production. It should be noted that **impaired mucosal blood flow and resultant mucosal ischaemia seem to be a major factor in critically ill patients.**

Two types of ulcer are classically eponymised:

■ Curling's ulcers associated with extensive burns
■ Cushing's ulcers associated with intracranial pathology and gastric acid hypersecretion

What measures have been employed to try and reduce the incidence of stress ulcers?

Adequate resuscitation is the main priority with **maximal oxygen transport to the gastric mucosa**. Attention should be paid to optimising cardiovascular variables and ensuring adequate gas exchange.

Other methods are used for stress ulcer prophylaxis:

■ **Enteral feeding**

■ **Sucralfate**   This is an aluminium salt of sulphated sucrose and is given in a dose of 1 g by NG tube, 6-hourly. It forms a paste at low pH which preferentially binds to areas of peptic ulceration, thereby providing a physical barrier to the effects of acid. Some investigators have demonstrated a reduction in the rate of nosocomial pneumonias in patients treated with sucralfate

■ **Antacids and**   These are the more traditional drugs used for stress
  H_2-antagonists   ulcer prophylaxis and may effectively reduce the risk of bleeding. There is, however, some concern that by increasing the pH of gastric contents, there is an increased risk of bacterial colonisation and subsequent nosocomial pneumonia

■ **Proton pump inhibitors**

A recent meta-analysis suggests that ranitidine is **ineffective** in the prevention of gastrointestinal bleeding in ICU patients and may increase the risk of pneumonia. The evidence for the use of sucralfate remains inconclusive.

References

Cook DJ *et al*. Risk factors for gastrointestinal bleeding in critically ill patients. *N Engl J Med* 1994; 330: 377–381

Eddleston JM *et al*. Prospective endoscopic study of stress erosions and ulcers in critically ill adult patients treated with either sucralfate or placebo. *Critical Care Medicine* 1994 22: 1949–1954

Eddleston JM *et al*. A comparison of the frequency of stress ulceration and secondary pneumonia in sucralfate- or ranitidine-treated intensive care unit patients. *Crit Care Med* 1991; 19: 1491–1496

Messori A *et al*. Bleeding and pneumonia in intensive care patients given ranitidine and sucralfate for prevention of stress ulcer: met-analysis of randomised controlled trials. *BMJ*, November 2000, Volume 321, number 7269, p1103–1106

Inhaled peanut

A 3-year-old boy has been admitted to casualty having inhaled a peanut 1 hour ago. You have been asked to assess him.

What are the symptoms of foreign body aspiration in a child?

There may be cough, choking, gagging and dyspnoea. If the obstruction persists the airway reflexes become fatigued resulting in an 'asymptomatic period'. Presentation after this time may be associated with airway erosion or infection. Peanuts can cause problems related to obstruction of the airway or secondary to the oil causing an inflammatory reaction.

What clinical signs would you look for?

- **Non-specific** signs of distress – tachycardia, tachypnoea and sweating
- Use of **accessory muscles** of respiration, **'tripod'** position
- Audible wheeze and stridor
- Examination of the chest may reveal **unilateral signs** such as increased percussion due to air trapping, wheeze and mediastinal shift or signs of lobar collapse. There may also be bronchial breathing and crackles depending on the duration of obstruction.

How would you manage the case?

Immediate assessment and initial management would follow the ABC principle. The need to intervene immediately is then determined. Most foreign body aspirations can wait until a suitable starvation time has elapsed providing the child is not too distressed. Dried beans or peas may require early intervention as they will expand with time.

Nebulised adrenaline (1:1000 solution at 0.5 ml/kg, max 5 ml) could be used as a holding measure to help reduce airway oedema (α effect). Heliox is also an option.

How would you anaesthetise this child having starved him?

- Consultant help should be available
- Calm environment
- Insertion of a cannula prior to induction would be ideal but may be determined by the likelihood of causing more distress to the child
- An **inhalational induction** with **sevoflurane in 100% oxygen** followed by endotracheal intubation to secure the airway would be appropriate
- The **surgeon should be on-hand**
- The ET tube may then be replaced with a **Storz ventilating bronchoscope**. A T-piece can then be connected to the side arm of the bronchoscope. A muscle relaxant may be used if necessary and lignocaine could be used to anaesthetise the airway
- In principle, positive pressure ventilation should be avoided until the peanut has been removed but it may be necessary if the bronchoscope lumen is narrow and the procedure is long

Why don't you want to use halothane?

Halothane has advantages and disadvantages over sevoflurane.

Advantages
- More potent
- Can achieve higher inhaled concentrations with halothane vaporisor (5 x MAC) compared with sevoflurane vaporisor (3 x MAC) – may make it easier to intubate without relaxant
- Less likely to lighten quickly resulting in laryngospasm

Disadvantages
- Longer time in stage two anaesthesia
- Slower onset than sevoflurane and slower return of airway reflexes
- Arrhythmias in children with hypoxaemia and hypercarbia

References
Hagberg CA. *Handbook of Difficult Airway Management*, 2000. Churchill Livingstone, Philadelphia, USA

Hatch DJ. New inhalation agents in paediatric anaesthesia, 1999. *BJA*, Volume 83 (1), p42–49

Mather S, Hughes D. *A Handbook of Paediatric Anaesthesia*, 2nd edition 1996. Oxford University Press, Oxford

Morton NS. Large Airway Obstruction in Children Parts 1 and 2, July and Sept 1999. CME core topic, *RCA Newsletter*

Intracranial pressure

What is normal intracranial pressure?

- Around 10 mmHg or less
- Sustained pressure of >15 mmHg is termed 'intracranial hypertension'
- Areas of focal ischaemia if ICP > 20
- Global ischaemia if ICP > 50
- Treatment usually considered if ICP > 20

> **Cerebral perfusion pressure:**
>
> **CPP = MAP – ICP** (or CVP if greater)
>
> - Normal CPP = 90–100 mmHg
> - Remember that adequate tissue perfusion is not just a function of CPP but depends on blood flow and oxygen content

What are the causes of raised intracranial pressure?

According to the **Munro–Kelly hypothesis** (1852) the contents of the cranium are not compressible. Any significant increase in the volume of brain tissue, blood or CSF within the cranium will lead to a rapid rise in intracranial pressure (ICP).

The causes of raised ICP may therefore be divided into three broad categories:

- **Brain**   Tumours
  Infection/abscess
  Oedema – three types: vasogenic, cytotoxic, interstitial
- **Blood**   Extradural
  Subdural
  Intracerebral
  Subarachnoid
  Venous congestion (e.g. cavernous sinus thrombosis)
- **CSF**   Outflow obstruction e.g. SAH, meningitis, tumours
  Increased production – choroid plexus papilloma (extremely rare!)
  Benign intracranial hypertension (usually young, obese women).

What are the symptoms and signs of raised intracranial pressure?

- **Symptoms**   Headache
  Vomiting
  Drowsiness
  Confusion
  Neck stiffness
  Seizures
- **Signs**   Depressed GCS
  Papilloedema (late sign)
  Cushing reflex (hypertension and bradycardia)
  Irregular respirations
  III and VI nerve palsies
- **Coning**   Two major types:
  1. **Tentorial** – the uncus of the temporal lobe compresses the brainstem on the contralateral side. This results in ipsilateral IIIn palsy, decreased GCS, Cushing reflex and decerebrate rigidity.
  2. **Cerebellar** – the medulla is compressed by the cerebellar tonsils passing through the foramen magnum resulting in Cheyne–Stokes breathing, sudden apnoea and neck stiffness.

What are the indications for ICP monitoring following head injury?

Some suggested indications include:

- GCS <8 with an abnormal CT scan
- Normal CT scan but two or more of the following factors
  Age >40
  Hypotension
  Unilateral posturing
  Bilateral posturing

How can you measure intracranial pressure clinically?

There are four methods commonly used via the skull and a lumbar approach via a CSF catheter.

1. Epidural catheter   Strain gauge transducer at tip or
                                 fibreoptically supplied light reflecting off a
                                 pressure-sensitive membrane
2. Subdural bolt or catheter   Prone to blocking and leak but less risk of
                                 infection than ventricular catheter
3. Ventricular catheter   Gold standard, accurate; CSF can be drained
                                 but risk of infection
4. Intraparenchymal catheter   Light reflecting pressure-sensitive membrane

The appropriate monitor will display the ICP and a waveform.

Lundberg waves:

A-waves   Sustained pressure waves (60–80 mmHg) every 5–20 minutes
          Life-threatening and represent cerebral vasodilatation in
          response to ↓CPP. Need urgent treatment
B-waves   Small and short lasting waves (10–20 mmHg) every 30–120
          seconds. Caused by fluctuations in CBV
C-waves   Small oscillations (0–10 mmHg), reflect changes in systemic
          arterial pressure

References

Deakin CD. *Clinical Notes for the FRCA*, 1998. Churchill Livingstone, Edinburgh
Hodgkinson V, Mahajan RP. The management of raised intracranial pressure. *RCA*, May 2000,
    Bulletin 1
Morgan GE, Mikhail MS. *Clinical Anaesthesiology*, 2nd edition, 1996. Appleton and Lange,
    Stamford, CT
Stone DJ et al. *The Neuroanaesthesia Handbook*, 1996. Mosby, St Louis, Missouri, USA

Ischaemic heart disease

Tell me about the principles of anaesthetising a patient with ischaemic heart disease (IHD).

> This is a question about myocardial oxygen supply and demand. You
> must relate the physiology to clinical practice.

The over-riding principle is to **avoid cardiac ischaemia** by ensuring that supply of oxygen to the myocardium always meets demand.

Supply

Supply of oxygen = Blood flow × Oxygen content

Blood flow is determined by:

- **Heart rate** determines coronary blood flow because diastole shortens with increasing heart rate
- **Aortic pressure** (particularly diastolic)

■ **Extravascular compression** of the coronary arteries (by a contracting ventricle). Blood flow in the coronary arteries is therefore greater in diastole. Compression during systole is greatest at the endocardium and this explains why this area is particularly susceptible to ischaemia. Blood flow in the left coronary artery may be reversed during systole
■ **Neurohumoral factors.** These are not of great importance. Autonomic nerve stimulation causes coronary vasoconstriction but this is offset by the vasodilatation that accompanies an increase in the myocardial metabolism
■ **Metabolic factors**. Coronary blood flow closely parallels myocardial metabolic activity

Oxygen content is determined by:

■ Haemoglobin concentration (but this alters viscosity and therefore blood flow!)
■ SaO_2
■ PaO_2

$$\text{Oxygen content} = (1.34 \times Hb \times SaO_2) + (0.003 \times PaO_2)$$

Demand

Determinants of myocardial oxygen demand are:

■ **Preload**, which determines LVEDP } Remember Laplace's law
■ **Afterload**
■ **Heart rate**
■ **Contractility**

In clinical practice this means avoiding:

■ **Hypoxia!**
■ **Hypotension** – especially diastolic
■ **Hypertension** – because it causes increased myocardial wall tension and thus further extravascular compression. It should be noted that pressure work increases myocardial O_2 consumption much more than volume work (increasing cardiac output) so hypertension must be avoided
■ **Tachycardia** – shortened diastole
■ **Stimulation of the autonomic nervous system**

A patient with ischaemic heart disease should be monitored for signs of ischaemia so that treatment can be instituted. **Monitoring** options include:

■ **CMV5**   Leads II and V5 together detect 95% of ischaemic events
■ **PAFC**
■ **TOE**
■ **Arterial line**   To detect hypotension quickly

What are the 'risk periods' during anaesthesia for patients with IHD?

The 'risk periods' are those times during the anaesthetic when the patient is more likely to develop **hypotension, hypertension and tachycardia**.

■ **Anxiety** pre-operatively causes hypertension and tachycardia
■ **Induction** can cause hypotension

- **Laryngoscopy** and **intubation** can cause hypertension and tachycardia as can
- **Surgical incision**
- **Extubation**
- **Pain** post-operatively
- **Hypoxia** is frequently responsible for ischaemic cardiac events post-operatively

Do you know any ways of modifying these responses?

- Premedication with anxiolytics, oxygen and usual cardiovascular medication
- Beta-blockers – recent interest in peri-operative beta-blockade and reduction in post-operative cardiac events. Wallace *et al* have shown that peri-operative atenolol for 1 week in patients at high risk for coronary artery disease significantly reduces the incidence of post-operative myocardial ischaemia. In addition there is a reduced risk of death for as long as 2 years after surgery
- Nitrates to induce coronary vasodilatation
- Cardiac stable induction agents (etomidate)
- Opioid-based anaesthetic technique
- Lignocaine spray to the cords (prior to intubation and extubation)
- Avoidance of cardiac depressant volatiles (e.g. halothane)
- Use of neuroaxial blocks (prevents stress response but beware hypotension)
- Post-operative oxygen

How do you assess cardiac risk?

- **History**
- **Examination** — These help guide further investigation
- **Investigations:**

	ECG	Arrhythmias predict peri-operative cardiac events
	Exercise ECG	Negative test correlates with low risk
	Ambulatory ECG	Can detect silent ischaemia
	Echocardiogram	Questionable value as a predictor of post-operative cardiac events
	Thallium scan	(with dipyridamole)
		Behaves like K^+
		Shows 'cold' spots
		No predictive value in most studies
	MUGA scan	Using technetium-99m
		Not of prognostic value
	Coronary	Expensive but useful
	Angiography	? Decrease in mortality rate afforded by CABG negated by risks of procedure itself

- **Scoring systems:** Clinical risk stratification indices
  Goldman (1977) – 9 factors. Maximum score = 53
  Detsky (1986) – additional factors to Goldman: MI at any time, unstable angina within 6 months, CCS angina Class III and IV, pulmonary oedema. Maximum score = 120.

Goldman index of cardiac risk in non-cardiac surgery

M.I. < 6 months	10
Age > 70 years	5
S3 or raised JVP	11
Important Aortic Stenosis	3
Rhythm other than sinus	7
> 5 VPBs per minute pre-op	7
Poor general medical state	3
pO$_2$ < 8 kPa	
pCO$_2$ > 6.7 kPa	
K$^+$ < 3.0 mmol/l	
HCO$_3^-$ < 20 mmol/l	
Urea > 18 mmol/l	
Creatinine > 260 μmol/l	
Chronic liver disease	
Bedridden	
Intraperitoneal, intrathoracic or aortic surgery	3
Emergency operation	4
Total	**53**

		Risk of cardiac death (%)
Class I	< 5 points	0.2
Class IV	> 25 points	56

■ **Studies:**   Rao *et al* (1983) Risk of recurrent peri-operative MI

         <3 months   = 5.7%

         >6 months   = 1.5%

Mangano (1990) Post-operative myocardial ischaemia is the most important predictor of adverse outcome

Shoemaker (1988) Patients able to increase their cardiovascular reserve pre-operatively (O$_2$ delivery/C.I.) do better

Diastolic hypertension is associated with increased risk of peri-operative complications

References

Berne RM, Levy MN. *Cardiovascular Physiology, 7th Edition*, 1997. Mosby, St Louis, Missouri, USA

Deakin CD. *Clinical Notes for the FRCA*, 1998. Churchill Livingstone, Edinburgh

Juste RN, Lawson AD, Soni N. Minimising cardiac anaesthetic risk: the tortoise or the hare? *Anaesthesia*, 1996, Volume 51, p255–262

Mangano DT. Assessment of the patient with cardiac disease – An anaesthesiologist's paradigm. *Anesthesiology*, 1999, Volume 91, p1521–1526

Wallace A *et al*. Prophylactic atenolol reduces postoperative myocardial ischemia. *Anesthesiology*, January 1998, Volume 88(1), p7–17

Jehovah's Witness ✓

What is the basis for Jehovah's Witnesses not accepting blood?

Since 1945, following a discussion in The Watchtower of Psalm 16 verse 4 (**'Their drink offering of blood I will not offer nor take up their names into my lips'**), Jehovah's Witnesses have refused transfused blood or blood products. The acceptance of blood is considered to be a violation of God's laws. This belief is further based on Genesis, Leviticus and Acts, all of which describe the prohibition of the consumption of blood.

> 'But flesh with the life thereof, which is the blood thereof, shall ye not eat' (**Genesis** 9: 3–4)
>
> 'ye shall eat the blood of no manner of flesh: for the life of the flesh is the blood thereof: whoever eateth it shall be cut off' (**Leviticus** 17: 10–16)
>
> 'That ye abstain from meats offered to idols, and from blood and from things strangled' (**Acts** 15: 28–29)

A reform movement now exists, called 'The Associated Jehovah's Witnesses for Reform on Blood', who are campaigning for the abolition of the blood transfusion policy.

What methods are available for minimising blood loss in a Jehovah's Witness?

Preoperatively
- Discussion with the patient regarding which (if any) blood products they are prepared to accept. Patients are frequently highly informed. At the patient's request a member of the Jehovah's Witness Hospital Liaison Committee may need to be involved. Similarly the patient will need to be seen on his or her own as well
- Full investigation of anaemia
- Involvement of a haematologist (consider pre-op erythropoietin or iron)
- Consultant involvement
- In obstetric cases, discuss the increased risk of hysterectomy (for PPH) and the use of an ultrasound scan to determine the placental site

Intraoperatively
- Positioning (avoiding venous congestion)
- Staged procedures
- Use of local or regional anaesthesia means the patient can stay awake and retract their prohibition if they feel the need
- Hypotensive anaesthesia – of proven use but important to weigh risks against benefits
- Haemodilution techniques – both hypervolaemic and normovolaemic
- Tourniquets

- Meticulous surgical technique/experienced surgeon
- Vasoconstrictor use
- Use of drugs that affect coagulation, e.g. tranexamic acid, aprotinin and desmopressin
- Cell-saver use will need to be discussed with the individual patient (Watchtower 1989)
- Balloon occlusion/ligation of arteries that supply the bleeding area

Postoperatively
- Minimal blood letting for laboratory testing
- ICU
- Erythropoietin
- GI bleeding prophylaxis
- Methods to decrease O_2 consumption: IPPV/barbiturates/neuromuscular blockers/hypothermia/hyperbaric oxygen therapy
- Perfluorocarbons
- Progesterone to decrease menstrual bleeding

Tell us about the legal aspects of giving blood to adults and children and consent validity

- It is **unlawful to administer blood to a patient who has refused it** by the provision of an Advanced Directive or by its exclusion in a consent form. To do so may lead to criminal proceedings
- Properly executed **Advance Directives must be respected** and special Jehovah's Witness consent forms should be widely available
- **A child's right to life is paramount and must be considered before the religious beliefs of his or her parents**
- If a child under 16 years old wishes to receive blood against their parents' wishes they must be shown to be **'Gillick competent'**
- In a **life-threatening emergency in a child** unable to give competent consent, **all life-saving treatment should be given**, irrespective of the patients' wishes
- In children of Jehovah's Witnesses under the age of 16 years the well being of the child is overriding. If the parents refuse to give permission for blood transfusion, it may be necessary to apply for a legal **'Specific Issue Order'**. This is a serious step that should be taken by two consultants
- In the case of children, application to the high court for a 'Specific Issue Order' should only be made when it is felt entirely necessary to save the child in an elective or semi-elective situation
- Except in an emergency, a doctor can decline to treat a patient if they feel pressurised to act against their own beliefs. The patient's management should be passed to a colleague

References
Kaufman L, Ginsberg R. *Anaesthesia Review 15*. Churchill Livingstone, 1999
Management of Anaesthesia for Jehovah's Witnesses, The Association of Anaesthetists of Great Britain and Ireland, 1999

Laparoscopic cholecystectomy

What are the problems associated with anaesthetising a patient for laparoscopic cholecystectomy?

The problems associated with laparoscopy are caused by:

- **Pneumoperitoneum**
- **CO_2** used as the insufflation gas
- **Positioning** on the table, i.e. reverse Trendelenburg
- **Surgical procedure** itself, i.e. cholecystectomy

These can be discussed in terms of their **physiological effects on the cardiovascular and respiratory systems** in particular. Other, less important changes are also seen in renal, metabolic and neuro-endocrine physiology.

Effects on the cardiovascular system

Haemodynamic changes are secondary to pneumoperitoneum, reverse Trendelenburg and the effects of the GA itself:

- **↓ Cardiac Index**   ↓ venous return by compression of IVC and reverse Trendelenburg position
  Paradoxically, CVP and PCWP ↑ – may be a result of central redistribution of blood or ↑ intrathoracic pressure
- **↑ SVR**   Aortic and splanchnic compression
  May also be due to humoral factors like catecholamines, PG's and vasopressin
- **↑ MAP**
- **Ischaemia**   Alterations in supply/demand
- **Arrhythmias**   Vagally mediated → A-V dissociation
                                   Nodal rhythm
                                   Sinus bradycardia
                                   Asystole
  Ventricular – related to high CO_2
- **Cardiac failure**

Effects on the respiratory system

These effects are mainly due to pneumoperitoneum and the use of CO_2 as the insufflation gas. Reverse Trendelenburg position actually attenuates some of the adverse effects (c.f. Trendelenburg for gynaecological surgery).

- **↓ FRC**   Diaphragmatic displacement cephalad
  ↓ chest wall dimension and muscular tone
  Changes in intrathoracic blood volume
  → **Atelectasis**
      Pulmonary shunting
      Hypoxaemia
- **↑ Airway pressures**   Peak airway pressure ↑ 6 cmH_2O
  May result in **barotrauma** or **pneumothorax**

- ↑ **Physiological dead space**
- ↓ **Total lung compliance**
- **CO$_2$ absorption**   ETCO$_2$ rises by 8–10 mmHg then plateaus at new level after about 40 minutes
  Respiratory acidosis with CVS consequences if not corrected
  Usually need 25% ↑ in minute volume
- **Endobronchial intubation**   The carina moves upwards during insufflation
  May also manifest as bronchospasm

Additional potential problems
- Acid aspiration
- Trocar injuries
- Venous gas embolism
- Bleeding
- Burns and explosions
- DVT

Reference
Coventry DM. Anaesthesia for laparoscopic surgery. June 1995. *J R Coll Surg Edinb, Volume* 40, p151–160

Latex allergy

A staff nurse presents for elective surgery and claims to have a history of possible latex allergy.

Who is at risk from developing latex allergy?

High-risk groups include:

- Patients with previous documented reactions
- Those exposed to repeated medical or surgical procedures involving the use of latex (especially bladder catheterisation)
- Health-care workers
- Patients with a history of atopy (may show cross-reactivity with certain foods especially banana, chestnuts and avocado)
- In spina bifida patients the prevalence may be as high as 60%

What types of allergy to latex do you know?

- Contact dermatitis   Type IV delayed hypersensitivity reaction to the chemical accelerators, anti-oxidants and stabilisers used in the manufacturing process
  T-cell mediated
- Anaphylaxis   Type I immediate hypersensitivity reaction to latex proteins in previously sensitised patients
  IgE mediated

How do you test for it?

Testing takes place 4–6 weeks after the reaction.

- **Skin-prick testing** Involves puncturing the skin with a thin needle through a drop of dilute antigen. The concentration of solution is important to avoid false negatives. There is a smaller risk of anaphylaxis than with intra-dermal testing
- **RAST** Radioallergoabsorbent testing is **less sensitive and more expensive** than skin-prick testing but **avoids the risk of anaphylaxis**

As there are many different latex proteins that may be implicated in the allergic response, a negative response to one antigen does not imply that the patient is not latex-sensitive. A strong clinical history suggestive of allergy is important.

How would you manage this case?

Having already been notified in advance, there is time to prepare the theatre environment and equipment necessary to undertake such a case. All theatre and ward staff should be aware of the necessary precautions to be taken. There should be a 'latex-free' box of equipment available and lists of equipment that:

1. Are latex-free
2. May be modified to be used
3. Must not be used at all

Premedication is controversial but may be given to patients who are considered to be very sensitive.

A suggested protocol for adults would be:

i.v. chlorpheniramine 10 mg 6 hourly
i.v. ranitidine 50 mg 8 hourly
i.v. hydrocortisone 100 mg 6 hourly
Salbutamol (inh/neb) for asthmatics

This would be given for 24 hours pre-operatively and at least 12 hours post-operatively. The patient should be first on the list and anaesthetised in a theatre unoccupied for at least 2 hours. The most important piece of equipment is latex-free gloves. All other equipment should be checked with the database in the 'latex-free' box.

Latex anaphylaxis:

- Reaction typically begins 30–60 minutes after the start of the procedure (c.f. anaphylactic reaction to i.v. drugs)
- Management as for anaphylaxis – think of latex-free environment as soon as is practical

---

Reference

Dakin MJ, Yentis SM. Latex allergy: a strategy for management. *Anaesthesia,* August 1998, Volume 53, p774–781

Lung cyst

A 62-year-old man presents for excision of a right-sided lung cyst.

What are the causes of lung cysts?

These may be congenital or acquired.

- **Congenital**   Bronchogenic
- **Acquired**   **Abscess** – e.g. tuberculosis, staphylococcal, klebsiella pneumonia, hydatid, septic pulmonary infarction, aspiration
  Tumour – cavitating primary bronchogenic or metastatic
  Bullae secondary to emphysema
  Bronchial obstruction following inhaled foreign body

This man has a right lower lobe abscess that requires resection. He has a history of emphysema. What are the important considerations when assessing this man?

The pre-operative assessment would concentrate on his respiratory function and exercise tolerance. Concomitant medical problems such as ischaemic heart disease are obviously also important. **Poor exercise tolerance, obesity and the presence of cardiovascular disease are strong indicators of a poor prognosis.**
    Routine investigations should include:

- Full blood count
- Electrolytes
- Clotting screen
- ECG
- Chest X-ray
- Pulmonary function tests
- CT/MRI of chest

An echocardiogram may also be indicated.
    Post-operative analgesia should be considered and discussed at this stage.

What would you expect the pulmonary function tests to show?

- ↓ FEV_1
- ↓ FVC
- ↓ FEV_1/FVC ratio
- Lung volumes may be normal or increased
- Transfer factor for carbon monoxide is low

What values for FEV_1 and FVC would you consider to be severe?

A predicted postoperative FEV_1 of less than 1 L will result in problems with sputum retention and less than 0.8 L is a contra-indication to lung resection.

What is maximum breathing capacity?

Maximum breathing capacity (MBC) is the product of maximum respiratory rate and tidal volume. The patient is asked to breathe in and out maximally for 15 seconds. The results are then multiplied by four to give the MBC. Normal is >60 L/min. Value of 25–50 L/min implies severe respiratory impairment.

What are the options for airway management in this man?

It is important to isolate the infected segment as far as possible by performing endobronchial intubation usually with a double-lumen tube. Re-usable tubes such as the Robertshaw and Carlens (carinal hook) or disposable tubes are suitable. The choice of induction may be influenced by the expected difficulty of intubation or the request by the surgeon to perform rigid bronchoscopy before the tube is inserted. Acceptable techniques include awake fibreoptic intubation, inhalational induction, rapid-sequence induction or even a conventional intravenous induction followed by a non-depolarising relaxant. In the latter technique, strong positive pressure should be avoided until the infected area is isolated. The patient should be positioned semi-sitting, ideally with the abscess-side down for induction.

How do you confirm correct placement of a double-lumen tube?

The procedure for a left-sided tube is as follows:

1. Inflate tracheal cuff (5–10 ml of air) → confirm bilateral breath sounds
2. Open tracheal lumen to air
3. Ventilate down bronchial lumen only (proximal clamp on catheter mount to tracheal lumen)
4. Inflate bronchial cuff (1–2 ml) until leak disappears (listen at open trachea lumen) and breath sounds heard only on left side
5. Unclamp catheter mount to tracheal lumen
6. Clamp catheter mount to bronchial lumen → confirm breath sounds heard only on right side
7. Unclamp both lumens

NB: The procedure may be altered in the case of a lung abscess where the infected lung needs to be isolated as soon as possible. In this case both cuffs may be inflated before any ventilation to reduce the risk of spillover into the good lung.

   The correct position should ideally be confirmed by the use of a fibreoptic bronchoscope. When it is passed down the tracheal lumen of a left-sided tube the carina should be visible with the bronchial cuff seen within the left main bronchus. The right main bronchus should also be visible and the origin of the right upper lobe bronchus may be seen.

What measures can be used to prevent or treat hypoxaemia during one-lung ventilation?

- ■ Administer 100% oxygen
- ■ Check position of DLT with fibreoptic scope
- ■ Oxygen may be insufflated into the collapsed lung via a suction catheter
- ■ PEEP to the dependent lung may expand collapsed alveoli
- ■ This may necessitate the application of CPAP to the collapsed lung to prevent a shift of blood flow secondary to the increase in pulmonary vascular resistance in the dependent lung
- ■ Intermittent two-lung ventilation if surgical access is compromised by the above manoeuvres
- ■ Clamping of the pulmonary artery supplying the collapsed lung may be required

Note that in general, ventilator settings used during two-lung ventilation need very little (if any) adjustment when one-lung ventilation is commenced.

What are the options for post-operative analgesia?

■ Intravenous opioids	Not ideal in patients with limited respiratory reserve
	Regional techniques are preferable
■ NSAIDs	
■ Epidural analgesia	May need supplementing with NSAIDs for shoulder-tip pain
■ Paravertebral block	May be less reliable than an epidural but fewer haemodynamic problems
■ Interpleural catheter	Placed by the surgeon
■ Intercostal blocks	By anaesthetist blind or by surgeon under direct vision

References

Coates M. A practical view of thoracic anaesthesia. *RCA Bulletin 6*, March 2001

Craft T, Upton P. *Key topics in Anaesthesia*, 2nd edition, 1995. Bios Scientific Publishers, Oxford

Kumar P, Clark M. *Clinical Medicine*, 3rd edition, 1994. Baillière Tindall, London

Morgan GE, Mikhail MS. *Clinical Anaesthesiology*, 2nd edition, 1996. Appleton and Lange, Stamford, CT

Pfitzner J, Peacock MJ, Tsirgiotis E, Walkley IH. Lobectomy for cavitating lung abscess with haemoptysis: strategy for protecting the contralateral lung and also the non-involved lobe of the ipsilateral lung. *BJA*, Nov 2000, Volume 85(5), p791–794

Malignant hyperthermia

Emergency scenarios you must know include:

- MH
- Cardiac arrest
- Anaphylaxis
- Failed intubation

How does malignant hyperthermia present?

- Rising end-tidal CO_2 is one of the first signs
- Tachycardia
- Arrhythmias
- Sweating
- Muscle rigidity
- Masseter spasm
- Temperature rise   Not necessarily an early sign
  Rate of rise 2–5°C/h

You mentioned a raised ETCO₂. How would you differentiate MH from other more common causes of a raised CO₂?

A raised $ETCO_2$ is not uncommon and may be due to:

- **Increased production**   Hypermetabolic states e.g. severe sepsis, thyrotoxic crisis, MH
  Reperfusion e.g. cross-clamp release
  Bicarbonate administration
- **Decreased excretion**   Decreased minute volume
- **Exogenous administration**   Laparoscopy
  Rebreathing

It is important to maintain a high index of suspicion of MH, being aware that it has a high mortality if left untreated (70%) – and indeed it is treatable. Therefore, if the $ETCO_2$ was high, one should exclude the more common causes of a raised $ETCO_2$ such as rebreathing or a reduced minute volume. The patient should be observed for sweating, flushing and signs of cardiovascular instability.
 Other differential diagnoses are:

- Malignant Neuroleptic Syndrome
- Ecstasy intoxication
- Inadequate anaesthesia or analgesia

How do you treat MH?

- **Stop administration** of any likely causative agents (volatiles)
- Change to a **vapour-free machine and circuit**. Use propofol/midazolam/opioids to keep the patient asleep if needed
- **Inform surgeons** and abandon surgery if possible

- **Summon help** – both a senior and further skilled anaesthetic assistance
- Give **100% O$_2$**
- **Hyperventilate** – increase minute volume by 2–3 times
- **Dantrolene** 1–10 mg/kg i.v. Initial dose is 1mg/kg. Repeat doses every 5 minutes until the reaction has stopped. Average dose needed to reverse MH crisis is 2.5 mg/kg. Assistance will be needed to draw this up, as it is slow to dissolve. Continue for 48 hours at a rate of 1–2 mg/kg every 4–6 hours
- **Measure core temperature**
- **Cool the patient** with ice/fan/tepid sponging/cold i.v. fluids and cold fluid into the bladder if practical. Cardiopulmonary bypass has been used
- Establish **invasive monitoring**: arterial line and CVP/PAFC
- Check K$^+$, CK and blood gases

What is the molecular basis for the clinical picture?

A genetic trait (mainly autosomal dominant) results in an error in skeletal muscle calcium control. The inborn error leads to a loss of control of calcium flux and an increase in the calcium concentration in the cytosol of skeletal muscle. The proposed site of action is the Ryanodine (a natural plant alkaloid) receptor, which spans the calcium-releasing channels on the sarcoplasmic reticulum and T-tubule.

The increase in intracellular free calcium results in the clinical picture of:

- Increased skeletal muscle contraction
- Increased skeletal muscle metabolism
- Glycolysis
- Rhabdomyolysis
- Uncoupling of oxidative phosphorylation

Dantrolene:

Vial containing orange powder
20 mg per vial
3 g of mannitol (to improve solubility)
Sodium hydroxide (to give pH of 9.5)
Reconstitute with 60 ml of water
Protect from light

Testing for MH susceptibility:

Halothane/Caffeine/Ryanodine contracture testing – with a strain gauge
Muscle biopsy from vastus lateralis
Divides into:
   MH susceptible – MHS
   MH negative – MHN
   MN equivocal – MHE
DNA testing is around the corner

References

Guidelines for the Management of a Malignant Hyperthermia Crisis. AAGBI, 1998

Hopkins PM. Malignant hyperthermia: advances in clinical diagnosis and management. *BJA* July 2000, Volume 85(1), p118–128

Massive blood transfusion

What is the definition of a massive blood transfusion?

Definitions do vary:

> Remember a couple of definitions and stick with them!

- **Replacement of total blood volume, with stored homologous bank blood, within 24 hours**
- Acute administration of more than 1.5 times the patient's blood volume
- A transfusion of half the blood volume per hour
- A transfusion greater than the total blood volume (10–20 units)
- > 6 units

What problems are associated with a massive transfusion?

> This is a very dry question and the answer is difficult to categorise. It will inevitably consist of a long list of facts.

Clotting abnormalities

Clotting abnormalities occur as a result of:

- **Blood loss** causing reduced levels of platelets, coagulation factors and inhibitors
- **Dilution** of these factors with volume replacement
  dilutional thrombocytopenia
  dilutional coagulopathy
  Only likely after a blood volume replacement with non-plasma fluid and red cells
- **DIC** may occur in 30% of patients who have a massive transfusion
  Lab results: Increased PT, APTT and FDPs
  　　　　　　　Decreased platelet count
  　　　　　　　Decreased fibrinogen
  DIC is generally due to hypoperfusion, etc. and not to transfusion itself

> **Storage**
>
> **Platelets** are unstable in stored blood at 4°C and the platelet count falls rapidly in blood stored for more than 24 hours.
>
> **Factor V** (50% after 14 days) and **VIII** (50% after 1 day) also lose activity on storage.

Biochemical complications

■ **Hyperkalaemia**	K^+ conc. in stored blood = 30 mmol/L after 3 weeks' storage
■ **Citrate toxicity**	Metabolised to bicarbonate in the liver resulting in metabolic alkalosis
	Patients who have liver disease or who are hypothermic are more prone to this >1 unit/5 min needed to overwhelm citrate metabolism
	Citrate binds to ionised calcium → hypocalcaemia
■ **Hypocalcaemia**	Causing decreased cardiac output – rare
■ **Acid–base disturbance**	Lactate from red cells
	Citric acid (the anticoagulant in donor blood)
	Acid–base balance depends on rate of blood administration, rate of citrate metabolism and the perfusion of the patient

Other problems

■ **Hypothermia**	Left shift of O_2 dissociation curve
	Platelet and clotting dysfunction
■ **Haemoglobin dysfunction**	Low temperature – left shift of O_2 dissociation curve
	Acidosis – right shift of O_2 dissociation curve
	Decreased levels of 2,3–DPG (especially after 14 days) – right shift of O_2 dissociation curve
■ **Haemolysis**	Due to osmotic fragility
■ **Incompatibility**	Errors occur more easily in extreme clinical situations
■ **Air embolism**	Potential hazard with the use of pressure bags
■ **Anaphylaxis**	3–5%

Delayed complications

■ **Disease transmission**	HIV/Hepatitis/Malaria/Bacteria → sepsis
■ **Immunosuppresssion**	Ca bowel recurrence, infection
■ **ARDS**	
■ **Pulmonary oedema**	

How would you manage a patient requiring a massive transfusion?

> **The aim is to restore:**
>
> ■ **Circulating volume** – mortality is increased with prolonged shock
> ■ **Oxygen carrying capacity** – packed cell volume > 0.20
> ■ **Haemostasis**
> ■ **Colloid osmotic pressure**
> ■ **Biochemical balance**

Points to mention are:

■ **ABC** approach	High flow O_2
	Large bore peripheral venous access with fluid warmers
	Keep the patient warm (warming blankets)
■ **Get help**	Senior assistance
	Haematologist – **communicate** with the lab!
	Surgical help – required to stop bleeding
Monitoring	Amount of blood loss – suction, weighing swabs
	Invasive arterial blood pressure
	CVP/PAWP
	Blood gases (repeated at intervals)
	Frequent clotting studies
	ECG
	Urinary catheter
	SaO_2
	$ETCO_2$
	Temperature (central and peripheral)
	A thromboelastograph may prove useful if available
■ **Equipment**	Rapid infusion device
	Cell saver
	Sengstaken–Blakemore tube
	MAST suit
■ **HDU/ICU**	
■ **FFP and platelets**	2 units of FFP and 5 units of platelets have been recommended in the past for every 8–10 units of blood transfused. However, **the need for supplements must be judged by clinical assessment and lab tests**
	FFP should be given if the PT is prolonged by more than 5 seconds
	Microvascular bleeding due to thrombocytopenia is more likely to occur if the platelet count is < 50 x 10^9/L. Treat with 6–8 units of platelets
■ **Cryoprecipitate**	Contains more **fibrinogen** and **Factor VIII**
	15 packs can be used to help treat **DIC**, which should be suspected if **thrombin time** is doubled

■ **Drugs**   **Aprotinin** – serine protease inhibitor → inhibits fibrinolysis
                       Tranexamic acid – antifibrinolytic agent that binds to
                       plasminogen and plasmin and interferes with their
                       ability to split fibrinogen
                       Desmopressin/vasopressin – affects circulatory
                       endothelial cells
                       Calcium chloride

Blood filters – a contentious issue

Designed to remove microaggregates:

■ **Micropore filters:** 2 types   Depth filters (impaction and adsorption)
  (20–40 μm)   Screen filters (direct interception principle)

  Problems: Impede blood flow, become blocked and activate complement
            Haemolysis and platelet depletion (depth filters)

■ **Standard blood filters** (170 μm)

References

Donaldson MDJ, Seaman MJ, Park GR. Massive blood transfusion. *BJA*, 1992, Volume 69, p621–630

Hewitt PE, Machin SJ. Massive blood transfusion. ABC of transfusion. *BMJ* Jan 1990, Volume 13,
   p107–109

Hoffbrand AV, Pettit JE. *Essential Haematology.* Blackwell Scientific Publications, Oxford, UK

Mitral stenosis

*A 56-year-old woman is listed for a laparoscopic cholecystectomy. She is
known to have mitral stenosis.*

What are the symptoms and signs of mitral stenosis?

Symptoms
■ Usually appear when the cross-sectional valve area is less than 2 cm^2
  (normal = 5 cm^2)
■ May be up to 20 years after the initial event which is almost always
  rheumatic fever
■ Recurrent bronchitis, dyspnoea, cough with bloodstained, frothy sputum
  (pulmonary oedema) and palpitations (secondary to atrial fibrillation).
  Eventually there is fatigue and peripheral oedema with the onset of right
  heart failure. There may also be symptoms related to systemic emboli and,
  rarely, a hoarse voice secondary to compression of the left recurrent
  laryngeal nerve by the enlarged left atrium.

Signs
■ Malar flush
■ Irregularly irregular pulse
■ Tapping, undisplaced apex beat (palpable first heart sound)

- Left parasternal heave
- On auscultation there is an opening snap (mitral valve) followed by a mid-diastolic, rumbling murmur localised to the apex
- There may also be signs of left and right heart failure and tricuspid regurgitation secondary to the back pressure from the left side

ECG
- If in sinus rhythm there will be biphasic P waves and signs of right heart strain
- Atrial fibrillation

Would you like any special investigations?

An **echocardiogram** would give an indication of the severity of the mitral stenosis in terms of the valve area and the pressure gradient across it.

Mitral stenosis is described as severe when the cross-sectional area is less than 1 cm^2.

What are the principles involved in anaesthetising this lady?

The problems associated with mitral stenosis will be complicated by the added effects of laparoscopy. This is a complex case as the haemodynamic changes associated with laparoscopy in a patient with mitral stenosis may make it very hazardous. The benefits of laparoscopic surgery would have to be weighed up against the risks of haemodynamic instability. An open cholecystectomy should be considered.

The principles involved in anaesthetising a patient with mitral stenosis are as follows:

- Establish **intra-arterial blood pressure monitoring.** Consider pulmonary artery catheter placement prior to induction although a pulmonary artery catheter has certain limitations in this situation. It may precipitate atrial fibrillation (if the patient is in sinus rhythm) with disastrous consequences and it may not reflect the true left ventricular end-diastolic pressure.
- **Avoid tachycardia** (which would reduce LV filling)
- **Maintain preload** without overdoing it. Hypovolaemia may lead to a marked reduction in cardiac output and overfilling could easily result in pulmonary oedema.
- **Avoid falls in SVR** – fixed cardiac output
- **Avoid increases in PVR:** hypoxia, hypercarbia, N$_2$O
- **Avoid vasodilators:** care with volatile agents
- **Maintain sinus rhythm** – be prepared to shock if patient goes into AF. Volatiles may lead to junctional rhythm with loss of atrial kick
- **Antibiotic prophylaxis** against endocarditis – BNF, probably amoxycillin and gentamicin in this case
- Post-operatively either HDU or ICU care would be appropriate

References
Deakin CD. *Clinical Notes for the FRCA*, 1998. Churchill Livingstone, Edinburgh
Morgan GE, Mikhail MS. *Clinical Anaesthesiology*, 2nd edition, 1996. Appleton and Lange, Stamford, CT

Mitral valve disease CXR

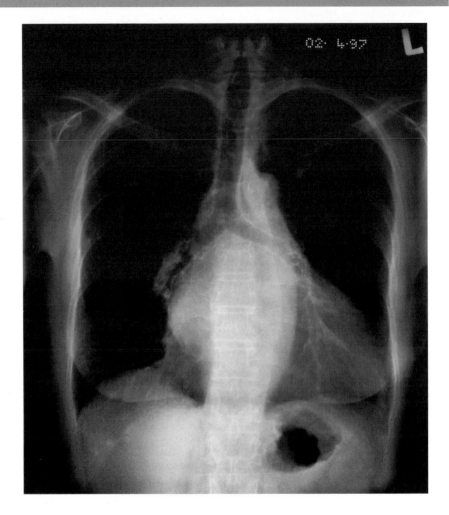

Have a look at this chest X-ray. What does it show?

- This is a PA chest X-ray of a female patient.
- The film is not rotated and is adequately penetrated.
- There is a **double heart border** on the right and straightening of the upper left heart border suggesting an enlarged left atrium. The **carina is splayed greater than 60°** and there is **upper lobe blood diversion**.
- These features suggest mitral stenosis. In addition there is cardiomegaly (CT ratio > 0.5) which only occurs in the presence of coexisting mitral regurgitation.
- The diagnosis is therefore **mixed mitral valve disease**.

What are the additional X-ray features that suggest severe, late disease?

These are the features of pulmonary hypertension and pulmonary oedema. In addition, the mitral valve annulus may be calcified.

> **X-ray features of pulmonary hypertension and oedema**
>
> ■ Pulmonary arteries prominent in perihilar regions but 'pruned' peripherally
> ■ Upper lobe blood diversion (mild venous hypertension)
> ■ Interstitial oedema (moderate) – fluid in fissures, pleural effusions and Kerley B lines
> ■ Alveolar oedema (severe) – pleural effusions, areas of consolidation and mottling of the lung fields

Myasthenia gravis

What is myasthenia gravis?

This is a rare condition characterised by **fatiguable weakness** classically affecting the **ocular, bulbar** and **proximal limb muscles**. There is **destruction of the acetylcholine receptor** protein at the (largely post-junctional) neuromuscular junction resulting in the failure of neuromuscular transmission. Serum **acetylcholine receptor antibodies** (polyclonal IgG) are present in 90% of generalised cases. It is twice as common in females, is associated with **thymoma in 10–15%** of cases and may be associated with other autoimmune conditions, e.g. thyrotoxicosis, rheumatoid arthritis, pernicious anaemia and SLE.

What is myasthenic syndrome?

This is a **paraneoplastic syndrome** also known as **Eaton–Lambert Syndrome** (ELS) characterised by proximal muscle weakness that typically affects the **lower extremities**. It is most commonly associated with **small-cell carcinoma** of the lung.

Can you compare and contrast the two conditions?

The two conditions differ in several ways.

■ **At a molecular level** Eaton–Lambert Syndrome results from a prejunctional defect in the quantal release of acetylcholine, which may be due to antibodies directed against calcium channels. Myasthenia gravis is due to a postjunctional defect as already described
■ **Clinically**, Eaton–Lambert Syndrome more commonly affects the lower limbs. It can also produce autonomic effects (hypotension, gastroparesis or urinary retention)
■ **Exercise** causes improvement in the weakness with Eaton-Lambert Syndrome ('second wind phenomenon') but worsening with myasthenia gravis. This can be easily demonstrated electrophysiologically (incrementing response as opposed to decrementing)

- **Anticholinesterases** do not cause an improvement with Eaton–Lambert syndrome. Instead, guanidine hydrochloride and 4-aminopyridine often help by enhancing Ach release by acting on calcium and potassium channels
- **Response to neuromuscular blockers.** ELS patients are sensitive to both depolarising and non-depolarising muscle relaxants. Myasthenia gravis patients are resistant to depolarising muscle relaxants

What problems does a patient with myasthenia gravis pose for the anaesthetist?

> Some form of categorising this question is worth learning. The problems of anaesthetising a myasthenic patient break down into the problems of:
>
> 1. Altered response to drugs, esp. muscle relaxants
> 2. The type of surgery being performed
> 3. Severity of disease
> 4. Co-existent medical (auto-immune) disease
> 5. Intercurrent medication – steroids, etc.
> 6. Exacerbation of disease
> 7. Post-op respiratory failure

- **Altered response to drugs**, especially muscle relaxants. The response to suxamethonium is unpredictable. Relative resistance (ED_{95} reported as 2.6 times normal), prolongation or a phase II block may be seen. Opioids or barbiturates may produce profound respiratory depression. Patients are often extremely sensitive to non-depolarising relaxants. Either avoid (patients can often be intubated with volatile alone) or use at about 1/10 of the usual dose. However, atracurium has been used without problems because of its rapid metabolism. A nerve stimulator must be used.
- **The type of surgery** being performed. With a thymectomy there is a risk of damage to the SVC and a risk of pneumothorax. Venous access in the lower limbs may be prudent. After trans-sternal thymectomy 50% of patients require post-operative ventilation
- **Severity of disease:**   Respiratory or bulbar muscle involvement?
  Increased risk of aspiration
  Arterial blood gases/CXR/PFTs will be needed to assess respiratory embarrassment
- **Co-existent auto-immune disease**
- **Current treatment** may include steroids, azathioprine, cyclophosphamide, cyclosporin and anticholinesterases (typically pyridostigmine which lasts about 3–4 hours). Medical treatment should be optimised. This may include plasmapheresis. There is debate about whether to reduce or stop anticholinergics before surgery. Patients are better off being slightly myasthenic rather than cholinergic. **Anticholinesterases** may cause:
  Increased vagal reflexes (? premedicate with atropine)
  The possibility of disrupting bowel anastomosis
  Prolonged action of ester-type local anaesthetics and suxamethonium (inhibition of plasma cholinesterase)

- **Exacerbation of the disease** may be caused by surgery, stress, infection, aminoglycosides, hypokalaemia and pregnancy.
- **Post-operative respiratory failure**. Increased risk with:
  - Disease duration > 6 years
  - Coexisting pulmonary disease
  - Vital capacity < 40 ml/kg
  - Pyridostigmine dose > 750 mg/day

Apart from needing surgery, how else may you be asked to help with the management of a myasthenic patient?

- **Intensive care management**
- Performance of an **edrophonium ('Tensilon') test** – distinguishing a myasthenic crisis from a cholinergic crisis. There is a risk of bradycardia and bronchoconstriction.

What is the difference between a myasthenic crisis and a cholinergic crisis?

- **A cholinergic crisis** is due to excessive administration of anticholinesterases and causes increased weakness with pronounced muscarinic effects:
  - Bradycardia
  - Salivation
  - Sweating
  - Small pupils
  - Lacrimation
  - Abdominal pain
  - Diarrhoea

  Edrophonium will exacerbate the weakness
- **A myasthenic crisis** is due to under treatment with anticholinesterases. Weakness will improve after administration of edrophonium

References
Baraka A. Anaesthesia and myasthenia gravis. *Canadian Journal of Anaesthesia* 1992, Volume 39(5), p476–486
Craft TM, Upton PM. *Key Topics in Anaesthesia*, 2nd Edition, 1995. Bios Scientific Publishers Oxford
Schady W. Myasthenia. *Current Anaesthesia and Critical Care*, 1997, Volume 8, p279–284

Myotonic dystrophy

A 35-year-old male patient with mild myotonic dystrophy presents for wisdom teeth extraction.

What is the underlying metabolic problem with this disorder?

It is an intrinsic muscle disorder. There is **delayed muscle relaxation due to abnormal closure of sodium/chloride channels** following depolarisation. This causes repetitive discharge and contraction.

What are the clinical features associated with myotonic dystrophy?

- **General**
  - Frontal balding
  - 'Lateral' smile
  - Muscle wasting – especially sternocleidomastoids, shoulders and quadriceps
  - Gonadal atrophy – infertility
  - Ptosis
  - Cataracts
  - Low serum IgG
- **Neurological**
  - Bulbar problems
  - Slurred speech
  - Dysphagia
  - Can lead to **aspiration**, a frequent cause of death
  - Decreased tone and reflexes with muscle wasting
  - Foot drop
  - Decreased IQ in 40%
- **Cardiac**
  - Conduction defects (1° heart block, bundle-branch block and widened QRS) – may need pacing
  - Increased QT_c and increased PR interval
  - Cardiomyopathy – cardiac failure
  - Mitral valve prolapse
- **Respiratory**
  - Respiratory muscle fatigue – poor cough – LRTI
  - Restrictive lung defect
  - Centrally mediated decreased ventilatory response to CO_2
  - Obstructive sleep apnoea
  - Chronic hypoxaemia
  - Cor pulmonale
- **Gastrointestinal**
  - Constipation
  - Delayed gastric emptying
- **Endocrine**
  - Diabetes
  - Hypothyroidism

What are the problems when anaesthetising these patients?

- **Undue sensitivity to anaesthetic drugs** (opioids, barbiturates and volatiles)
- **Precipitation of myotonia** by:
  - Anaesthetic and surgical interventions
  - Diathermy
  - Cold (monitor temperature)
  - Pregnancy (atonic uterus and PPH also reported)
  - Shivering (avoid high volatile concs)
  - Suxamethonium
  - Non-depolarising muscle relaxants
  - Anticholinesterase drugs
  - K^+ containing solutions
  - Exercise

- **Cardiovascular and respiratory problems** – especially the risk of aspiration
- **Control of blood sugar** as many of these patients have diabetes
- **Drug interactions** with concomitant drug treatment   Phenytoin
                                                                Quinine
                                                               Procainamide
- **Presentation** may be late on in the disease (2nd–4th decade) and the disease may therefore present undiagnosed to the anaesthetist

NB: No proven link with malignant hyperthermia.

What anaesthetic techniques can be used?

- **Pre-operatively** these patients should have:
An ECG (24 hour if appropriate)
Full blood count, urea, electrolytes (**NB:** K$^+$) and a blood sugar
Pulmonary function tests
Arterial blood gases
Chest X-ray
- **Premedication** – respiratory depressants should be avoided
Antacids are advisable
- **Invasive monitoring** would be appropriate (arterial line/CVP/PAFC) if there is a history of arrhythmias or cardiomyopathy
- **Temperature** must be monitored and attention paid to keeping the patient warm. Warming mattresses and warmed i.v. fluids
- **Induction and maintenance**. Propofol has been shown to be safe. Extreme caution with dosing. Intubation is necessary to protect against aspiration. High concentrations of volatiles should be avoided as they can cause shivering and hence myotonia
- **Regional techniques** will avoid the use of general anaesthetic drugs that can precipitate myotonia. Nerve blockade will not however prevent the myotonic reflex. Local anaesthetic infiltration into the *muscle* can prevent this reflex
- If a **muscle relaxant** must be used then the agent of choice would be atracurium. Neuromuscular block monitoring is essential
- **Post-operatively**, HDU or ICU care should be considered. Early feeding should be avoided due to the possibility of aspiration

References

Goldstone JC, Pollard BJ. *Handbook of Clinical Anaesthesia,* 1996. Churchill Livingstone, Edinburgh
Morgan GE, Mikhail MS. *Clinical Anaesthesiology*, 2nd edition, 1996. Appleton and Lange, Stamford,CT
Russell SH, Hirsch NP. Anaesthesia and myotonia. *BJA*, 1994, Volume 72, p210–216

Obesity

A 40-year-old female (weight = 120 kg, height = 155 cm) is on your list for an abdominoplasty.

How can you classify obesity?

There are numerous classification systems for categorising the relationship between height and weight. The two commonest are:

- The **body mass index** (BMI) is a useful method and is calculated by
  BMI = weight (kg)/height squared (m2)
    - 22–25 is normal
    - 25–30 is considered overweight
    - >30 is obesity
    - >35 is morbid obesity
- The **Broca Index** is another method and has different formulas for males and females.
    - Normal weight (kg) for males = height (cm) – 100
    - Normal weight (kg) for females = height (cm) –105

This lady's BMI is 49, which would define her as morbidly obese.

What are the problems that her obesity may pose for anaesthesia?

> There are two approaches to this question. The one you choose will be a combination of personal choice and the way in which the question is asked.
>
> 1. A **body systems** approach – describing the pathophysiology of each system. The danger with this method is that it is easy to omit practical problems, e.g. cannulation, positioning and monitoring
> 2. A more practical, **chronological approach** listing the problems encountered from the pre-operative, through to the post-operative period

Cardiovascular
- **Increased blood volume and cardiac output** leading to cardiomegaly, left ventricular hypertrophy (therefore reduced compliance and diastolic function) and a potential for left ventricular failure.
- **Hypertension** and **ischaemic heart disease** are common
- **Venous access** can sometimes be difficult
- **Thromboembolism** risk is increased

Respiratory
- **Increased work of breathing**
- **Reduced compliance** (both chest wall and lung) and **reduced FRC** will predispose to atelectasis, increased shunt and hypoxia. These patients must be preoxygenated as they desaturate much quicker than non-obese (3–5 times)

- Pulmonary vasoconstriction, **pulmonary hypertension** and right ventricular hypertrophy
- Oxygen consumption and carbon dioxide production are increased
- **Obstructive sleep apnoea** is relatively common and 5% have **Pickwickian Syndrome** in which there is a loss of the sensitivity to hypercarbia resulting in a combination of **hypoxia, cor pulmonale and polycythaemia**
- There is a higher incidence of **difficult laryngoscopy**

This presents the anaesthetist with a patient who may be difficult to bag-mask ventilate, difficult to intubate and will desaturate quickly.

Gastrointestinal
- **Increased acidity and volume** of gastric contents
- **Hiatus hernia** and **gallstones** are common associations
- **Increased intra-abdominal pressure**
- There is a higher risk of **regurgitation and aspiration** requiring rapid sequence induction if a difficult airway is not anticipated
- Tracheal extubation should be undertaken with the patient awake

Endocrine
- There is an association with **glucose intolerance**

Morphological
- **Positioning**
- **Transferring**
- **Monitoring** (arterial line may be needed if NIBP is problematic)

How would you assess this lady's airway?

Incidence of difficult intubation in morbidly obese is around 13%.

Altered anatomy: Increase in soft tissue
Reduced head and neck mobility
Large tongue
Short neck
Large breasts
Anterior larynx
Restricted mouth opening

History
- Symptoms of obstructive sleep apnoea including snoring and daytime hypersomnolence
- Previous anaesthetic charts should be reviewed to determine if there were problems with airway maintenance in the past

Examination
- Assessment of head and neck movement
- Mouth opening

- Mandibular movement
- Thyromental distance
- Nostril patency

Investigations
- Indirect laryngoscopy may be useful
- Radiology

Tell me how you would anaesthetise this lady.

> There is no one right answer to this question. Whichever method is chosen should be systematic and start with history, examination and investigations. Conduct of anaesthesia, including premedication and postoperative management, should then be discussed. The examiner may stop you and jump to an issue they wish to explore.

Having taken a history, examined the patient and performed appropriate investigations, consideration should be given to premedication. Antiemetics and sodium citrate may be prescribed and an anticholinergic agent should be given if fibreoptic intubation is considered.

If a difficult intubation is not anticipated the patient should be preoxygenated for at least 3 minutes and a rapid sequence induction performed with cricoid pressure. All difficult airway adjuncts should be immediately available. Once the airway is secured with an endotracheal tube the patient should be ventilated. Compared to non-obese patients, a higher FiO_2 and the addition of PEEP may be required to help prevent basal atelectasis. However, the addition of PEEP may adversely affect venous return and cardiac output.

A combination of general and regional anaesthesia has many advantages but:

- Regional blocks can be technically difficult as anatomical landmarks may be obscured. Longer needles may be necessary
- Epidural local anaesthetic dose requirements are reduced as the volume of the epidural space is reduced

Important postoperative considerations include:

- Extubate awake, sitting up
- HDU care, may need CPAP
- Oxygen and oximetry
- Obstructive sleep apnoea is most common *some days* after surgery
- Adequate analgesia to allow deep breathing/coughing
- Physiotherapy
- DVT prophylaxis

References
Adams JP, Murphy PG. Obesity in anaesthesia and intensive care. *BJA*, July 2000, Volume 85(1), p91–108
Brodsky JB. Morbid obesity. *Current Anaes and Crit Care*, 1998, Volume 9, p249–254

Pacemakers

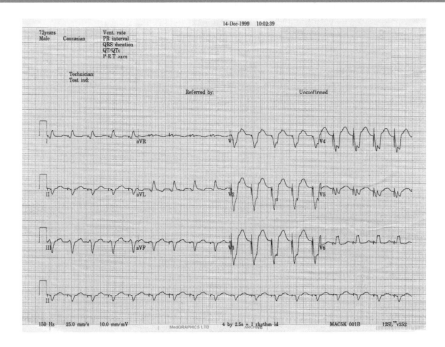

Have a look at this ECG

The ECG shows paced rhythm from a ventricular pacemaker with a rate of approximately 100 bpm. The QRS complexes are broad and bizarre-looking in keeping with the abnormal pathway through slower conducting ventricular tissue.

How are pacemakers classified?

There is a **five letter code** that describes the characteristics of each permanent pacemaker. The first three letters are the most important.

Letter

I Chamber paced	O = None
	A = Atrium
	V = Ventricle
	D = Dual
II Chamber sensed	O = None
	A = Atrium
	V = Ventricle
	D = Dual
III Response to sensed	O = None
information	T = Pacemaker triggered
	I = Pacemaker inhibited

D = Dual (ventricular-sensed events lead to inhibition but atrial-sensed events trigger ventricular output)

IV Programmability, rate modulation	The ability of the pacemaker to alter the pacing rate in response to physiological variables such as increased activity, respiration or blood temperature (various letters assigned)
V Anti-tachycardia functions	O = None P = Anti-tachycardia pacing S = Shock, i.e. cardioversion/defibrillation D = Dual

Thus, a pacemaker with the code **DDIRO** represents a dual-chambered pacemaker that is inhibited when it senses intrinsic electrical activity, possesses a rate-response facility and has no automatic shock facility.

What is the anaesthetic management of a patient who is fitted with a pacemaker and requires surgery?

The main peri-operative problems in a patient with a permanent pacemaker are due to the effects of anaesthetic agents, altered physiology and surgical diathermy.

Pre-operative assessment
Usual anaesthetic assessment plus:

- **Establish the original indication** for inserting the pacemaker, what type it is, when it was last checked and information about any programmed functions it may have
- Look for symptoms that may suggest problems with pacing, e.g. syncope or palpitations
- Pacemakers with rate-responsive or anti-tachycardia modes should probably have them deactivated pre-operatively
- **Check pacemaker function:** ECG
  If the intrinsic rate is higher than that set on the pacemaker then a Valsalva manoeuvre may be employed to check function
  CXR will identify number and integrity of leads
- **Check electrolytes** – especially K^+ Hypokalaemia → loss of capture
  Hyperkalaemia → ventricular irritability
- Acid–base disturbances, some antiarrhythmic drugs, digoxin toxicity and hypothermia may influence capture. These should be addressed and corrected if necessary.
- If in doubt get a cardiology opinion – may require temporary pacing

Intra-operative management
- Appropriate monitoring based on pre-op assessment
- An alternative means of pacing must be immediately available: external, transvenous or oesophageal

- Care at induction – may result in stimulation or inhibition of the pacemaker due to alterations in myocardial conduction or sensed muscular contractions (e.g. etomidate or suxamethonium) depending on the pacemaker program
- Volatile agents also alter the pacing threshold and in high concentration will increase the risk of arrhythmias and ectopics
- Avoid hypoxaemia and hypercarbia – ectopics and arrhythmias
- Rate-responsive pacemakers may induce a tachycardia in response to a high respiratory rate set on the ventilator
- **Diathermy** The use of diathermy may reprogram the pacemaker, cause microshock or induce VF. Bipolar should be used if possible or if unipolar is essential the plate should be placed as far away from the heart as possible. Short bursts followed by long pauses should be used.
- **Magnets** In general should not be used. If placed over a programmable pacemaker in the presence of electromagnetic interference (e.g. diathermy) there may be unpredictable reprogramming.
  The magnet may also initiate a 'threshold test' whereby the output current gradually decreases until failure of capture occurs! Although the 'magnet rate' is usually written on the packaging for each pacemaker, most anaesthetic references now recommend that magnets are not used.
- Peripheral nerve stimulators may interfere with pacing
- If DC cardioversion is required the paddles should be placed perpendicular to the direction of the pacing wire. The box is designed to protect itself by diverting current away from the internal circuitry which may then pass down a damaged lead resulting in burns
- Isoprenaline may be required as a holding measure while emergency pacing is achieved in the event of pacemaker failure

Post-operatively
- Pacemaker function should be checked at the pacemaker clinic

References
Bennett DH. *Cardiac Arrhythmias*, 4th edition, 1994. BH publishing, Oxford
Bourke M. The patient with a pacemaker or related device. *Can J Anaesth*, 1996, Volume 43(5), pR24–R32
Deakin CD. *Clinical Notes for the FRCA*, 1998, Churchill Livingstone, Edinburgh
Morgan GE, Mikhail MS. *Clinical Anaesthesiology*, 1996. Appleton and Lange, Stamford, CT

Penetrating eye injury

You are asked to anaesthetise a 15-year-old girl who sustained a penetrating eye injury 1 hour ago. She is fit and well but had fish and chips just prior to her injury.

What are the issues here?

There are two major and conflicting priorities in this case.

1. The need to minimise the risk of aspiration in a patient requiring emergency anaesthesia with a full stomach
2. The need to avoid a rise in intra-ocular pressure (IOP)

What are the determinants of intra-ocular pressure?

- Normal IOP is 12–20 mmHg.
- The eye can be thought of in a similar way to the skull. If any of the contents of this 'rigid' sphere (such as blood or aqueous humour) increase then the IOP will increase.
- Raised IOP may be caused by direct pressure on the eye, raised CVP, hypertension, hypercarbia, hypoxia, coughing, straining or alterations in production/drainage of aqueous humour.
- When the globe is open the IOP is equal to atmospheric pressure, therefore anything that would normally lead to raised IOP will lead to extrusion of intra-ocular contents.

How do induction agents alter IOP?

Most reduce IOP with the exception of ketamine, which may cause an increase via hypertension. (Ketamine may also cause nystagmus and blepharospasm.)

How do volatile anaesthetics alter IOP?

All modern inhalational agents reduce IOP in proportion to the depth of anaesthesia. The fall in BP with increasing depth of anaesthesia reduces choroidal blood volume and relaxes the extra-ocular muscles. The pupillary constriction aids aqueous drainage.

How do muscle relaxants alter IOP?

Non-depolarising agents reduce or do not alter IOP.
  Suxamethonium increases IOP by around 5–10 mmHg for 5–10 minutes.

Why does suxamethonium have this effect?

The extra-ocular muscles have a more prolonged contraction compared with other skeletal muscles due to their innervation by multiple neuromuscular junctions ('en-grappe' = bunch of grapes) on each muscle fibre.

How will you manage this case?

Local anaesthesia is not suitable, as IOP will be raised by injecting around the globe. An assessment of the degree of urgency should be made with the surgeon to delay until an adequate starvation time has elapsed if possible.

The surgeon is jumping up and down to do the case straight away.

What will you do?

■ Delay surgery
■ Rapid sequence induction
■ Obtund response to suxamethonium/laryngoscopy/intubation

This is **not a life-threatening emergency** and therefore the risk of aspiration should be minimised by delaying surgery and giving metoclopramide, ranitidine and sodium citrate to help empty the stomach and raise the pH of any remaining contents.

The patient will require a **rapid sequence induction** with cricoid pressure. The main issue here is the use of suxamethonium. If the intubation looks straightforward then rocuronium could be considered but if there is any doubt then the protection of the airway should come first. In a study of RSI using suxamethonium in 228 patients with penetrating eye injury there was no loss of vitreous through the eye wound (Libonati et al 1985).

Fentanyl (3–5 μg/kg), **alfentanil** (20 μg/kg) or **lignocaine** (1.5 mg/kg) could be used to obtund the hypertensive response to laryngoscopy.

Recently, **remifentanil** (1 μg/kg immediately prior to induction) has also been shown to effectively obtund the IOP response to suxamethonium and intubation.

Attention should be given to general measures to prevent a rise in IOP. These are similar to those used in the management of raised ICP.

The patient should be extubated awake as protection of the airway takes priority.

If IOP increases intra-operatively what would you do?

■ Look for a cause and treat
■ Other therapeutic measures

It is important to ensure adequate depth of anaesthesia and analgesia. Hypercarbia and hypoxia should be addressed, as should any obstruction to venous flow. Mannitol (0.5 g/kg) or acetazolamide (500 mg) could be considered.

What is the oculo-cardiac reflex and how is it managed?

It may occur following pressure on the eyeball, traction on the extra-ocular muscles, pain or raised IOP. There may be bradycardia, nodal rhythm, ectopic beats, sinus arrest or even ventricular fibrillation.

The afferent passes via the ophthalmic division of the trigeminal nerve to the sensory nucleus in the fourth ventricle. The efferent is supplied via the vagus.

Management involves informing the surgeon, ensuring adequate depth of anaesthesia and analgesia and administering atropine or glycopyrrolate if it persists.

References

Craft TM, Upton PM. *Key Topics in Anaesthesia*, Second edition, 1995. Bios Scientific Publishers, Oxford

Deakin CD. *Clinical Notes for the FRCA*, 1998. Churchill Livingstone, Edinburgh

Libonati MM, Leahy JJ, Ellison N. The use of succinylcholine in open eye surgery. *Anaesthesiology* 1985, Volume 62, p637–640

Morgan GE, Mikhail MS. *Clinical Anaesthesiology*, 2nd edition, 1996. Appleton and Lange, Stamford, CT

Ng H-P, Chen F-G, Yeong S-M, Wong E, Chew P. Effect of remifentanil compared with fentanyl on intraocular pressure after succinylcholine and tracheal intubation. *BJA* 2000, Volume 85(5), p785–787

Pneumonectomy

A 67-year-old man is listed for a right pneumonectomy for carcinoma of the lung.

What histological types of bronchial carcinoma are there?

- Squamous   35%
- Adenocarcinoma   20%
- Large cell   19%
- Small (oat) cell   25%

What are the symptoms and signs of bronchial carcinoma?

The commonest **symptoms** are cough, haemoptysis and dyspnoea followed by chest pain, wheeze and weight loss.

Signs include clubbing, wheeze, stridor and supraclavicular lymph nodes.

The signs of the *complications* of bronchial carcinoma are varied and can be categorised into:

- **Intrathoracic**   Pleural effusion
  SVC obstruction
  RLN palsy
  Phrenic nerve palsy
  Horner's syndrome
  Pericarditis, cardiac arrhythmias (especially AF)
  Rib erosion
- **Non-metastatic**   Ectopic hormone secretion e.g. ADH/ACTH from oat cell tumours

Neuromuscular e.g. mixed sensorimotor peripheral neuropathy, encephalopathy, proximal myopathy, Eaton–Lambert (myasthenic) Syndrome and polymyositis

Haematological e.g. anaemia, polycythaemia, bleeding disorders

Weight loss

Hypertrophic pulmonary osteoarthropathy

Thrombophlebitis migrans

■ **Metastatic**   Brain, bone, liver, adrenals, skin, kidney

What are the risk factors for developing a bronchial carcinoma?

The biggest risk factor is cigarette smoking but others include:

■ Increasing age
■ Male > female
■ Asbestos exposure
■ Radiation

What are the important considerations in your pre-operative assessment?

There are now guidelines on the selection of patients with lung cancer for surgery. These assess a patient's fitness for surgery based heavily on age, pulmonary function and cardiovascular fitness. Risk is stratified into minor, intermediate and major.

Age

Perioperative morbidity for lung cancer surgery increases with age. Mortality rates for pneumonectomy average 14% in the elderly (higher than in younger patients) and therefore age should be a factor in assessing suitability for pneumonectomy.

Pulmonary function

1. If FEV_1 > 2.0 L then no further respiratory function tests are required
2. If FEV_1 < 2.0 L then *postoperative* FEV_1 and TL_{CO} need to be estimated and compared to predicted values for normal patients

Estimated postoperative FEV_1 > 40% predicted
Estimated postoperative TL_{CO} > 40% predicted   } average risk
Saturation > 90% on air

Estimated postoperative FEV_1 < 40% predicted
Estimated postoperative TL_{CO} < 40% predicted   } high risk

All others – exercise testing

High risk patients need formal multidisciplinary discussion and consideration of alternative treatment.

Cardiovascular fitness

There is little specific information relating to the cardiac risks of patients who are undergoing pneumonectomy and most data surround the 'non-cardiac surgery' group. Clinical predictors of increased perioperative cardiovascular risk include:

- Major
  - Recent MI
  - Grade 3 or 4 angina (Canadian Cardiovascular Society)
  - Decompensated CCF
  - Significant arrhythmias
  - Severe valvular disease
- Intermediate
  - Grade 1 or 2 angina (CCS)
  - Prior MI
  - Compensated CCF
  - Diabetes mellitus
- Minor
  - Advanced age
  - Abnormal ECG
  - Rhythm other than sinus
  - Low functional capacity
  - History of stroke

Other considerations preoperatively are weight loss, nutritional status and other medical co-morbidities.

References

British Thoracic Society. Guidelines on the selection of patients with lung cancer for surgery. *Thorax*, 2001, Volume 56, p89–108

Kumar PJ, Clark ML. *Clinical Medicine*, 2nd edition, 1990. Baillière Tindall, London

Pneumothorax

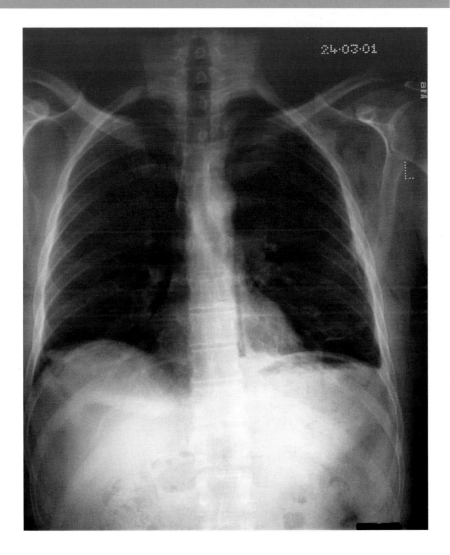

What does this chest X-ray show?

This is a PA chest X-ray of a male patient. There is a small left-sided pneumothorax with some associated surgical emphysema seen particularly overlying the scapular region. There is no obvious cause such as a central line or fractured rib.

What are the causes of pneumothorax?

- **Trauma**
  Penetrating chest injury
  Fractured rib
- **Spontaneous**
  Usually young thin males
  Associated with Marfan's syndrome

	Ascent in aeroplanes
	Wind instrument players!
■ **2° to underlying chest disease**	Pneumonia/TB/lung abscess
	Diffuse lung disease
	Emphysematous bulla
	Carcinoma
	Asthma
■ **Iatrogenic**	Central line insertion
	IPPV

What are the symptoms and signs of a pneumothorax?

■ Symptoms	Shortness of breath
	Pleuritic chest pain
■ Signs	Decreased expansion
	Increased percussion note
	Decreased breath sounds
	Decreased SaO_2

Tension pneumothorax

Features as above plus

- ■ Contralateral mediastinal shift
- ■ Cardiovascular collapse

Note that there may be few physical signs if the pneumothorax is small.

How do you insert an intercostal drain?

- ■ Establish i.v. access
- ■ Prepare the insertion site – anterior axillary line in the 5th intercostal space
- ■ Infiltrate with local anaesthetic (10–20 ml of 1% lignocaine)
- ■ 2–3 cm incision parallel to and just superior to the rib
- ■ Blunt dissection down to the pleura with artery forceps and finger
- ■ Puncture the pleura with blunt forceps (a patient on IPPV should be disconnected from the ventilator prior to this manoeuvre)
- ■ Finger sweep into the pleural cavity to ensure that the lung is not adherent to the insertion site
- ■ Clamp the proximal end of the tube and insert without the trocar
- ■ Direct the tube towards the apex (towards the base for fluids – not essential)
- ■ Connect the tube to an underwater drainage system
- ■ Suture in place and apply dressing
- ■ Obtain a chest X-ray

Tell me about underwater seals?

The intercostal tube is placed with the tip lying 2–3 cm under the surface of the water. This provides a one-way valve system for the drainage of air. Fluid will drain with gravity. The underwater seal system needs to be kept below the level of the patient so that fluid does not drain back into the chest under hydrostatic pressure.

Spontaneous breathing

On inspiration, a negative intrapleural pressure is created (around –8 cm of water in tidal breathing). The fluid level in the tube will therefore rise. If the underwater seal was not present, air would be sucked into the pleural cavity. On expiration, intrapleural pressure will become positive if chest wall pressure exceeds alveolar pressure. If this occurs then air will be expelled via the drain.

IPPV

On inspiration, a positive intrapleural pressure is created which results in the drainage of air. On expiration, the intrapleural pressure will still be positive if there is PEEP applied to the lungs and therefore air will still drain.

A potential problem may arise when using traditional chest drain bottles to drain fluid and air simultaneously. As the fluid level in the bottle (and thus the submerged end of the tube) rises, a higher positive intrapleural pressure will be required to drain air. Hence, the lung may not fully re-expand and in the case of a persistent leak a tension pneumothorax could develop (or may just drain at a higher pressure). Modern chest drain bottles are now designed to maintain the submerged end of the intercostal drain at less than 2–3 cm below the level of the fluid.

Tell me about suction applied to intercostal drains?

Suction can be used to increase the drainage from the pleural space. Only high-volume, low-pressure pumps should be used. A pressure of 10–20 cmH$_2$O is adequate for a pneumothorax. Low-volume, high-pressure pumps are dangerous and should not be used. The low volume displacement may not be able to cope with large air leaks, resulting in tension. High pressure may result in damage to the visceral surface of the lung.

When would you clamp an intercostal drain?

This is controversial. Some authorities state that there are no indications to clamp a drain. Some points to note are:

- Never clamp a bubbling chest drain
- Drains should not be clamped during transfer
- Drains should be clamped after a pneumonectomy. If they are not then catastrophic mediastinal shift can occur. Every hour the drain should be unclamped briefly to look for significant postoperative bleeding
- Large effusions can drain rapidly resulting in re-expansion pulmonary oedema (may be unilateral). This can cause chest discomfort and tightness and has resulted in death. Clamping the drain for a period of time (4 hours has been suggested) after removing 1–1.5 litres of fluid allows the lung to re-expand in a controlled manner

References

ATLS Course for Physicians, 1993. American College of Surgeons

Hall M, Jones A. Reducing morbidity from insertion of chest drains. (Letter) *BMJ,* August 1997, Volume 315, p313

Harriss DR, Graham TR. Management of intercostal drains. *British Journal of Hospital Medicine,* June 1991,Volume 45, p383–386

Hyde J, Sykes T, Graham T. Reducing morbidity from chest drains. *BMJ,* March 1997, Volume 314, p914–915

Kumar P, Clark M. *Clinical Medicine,* 3rd edition, 1994. Baillière Tindall, London

Oh TE. *Intensive Care Manual,* 4th edition, 1997. BH publishing, Oxford

Skinner D, Driscoll P, Earlam R. *ABC of Major Trauma.* 1991. BMJ publishing

Post-herpetic neuralgia

What do you understand by the term neuralgia?

This is simply a mononeuropathy of a named nerve.

Can you tell me something about the pathogenesis of post-herpetic neuralgia?

This can develop after an acute herpes zoster infection. There is reactivation of a dormant varicella zoster virus (chickenpox). The infection causes nerve fibre damage by inflammation and ischaemia in both sensory and motor (usually subclinical) nerves. These lesions are at the dorsal root, dorsal root ganglion and dorsal horn.

What are the clinical features?

The initial herpes zoster is painful and has a variable time course. There is no set definition of post-herpetic neuralgia, but some authors use the presence of pain persisting at 1 month as diagnostic.

The syndrome occurs predominantly in patients over the age of 50 and is normally isolated to a single dermatomal segment, frequently unilateral. Thoracic dermatomes and the ophthalmic division of the trigeminal nerve are common sites.

The pain itself is severe with constant aching, burning or itching. There may be superimposed bouts of stabbing pain. Pigmentation and scarring may also occur.

What are the treatment options available?

- ■ **Tricyclic antidepressants**
  These currently seem to be the most effective drugs used. Amitriptyline is commonly used as first line and changed or added to if not wholly effective.
- ■ **Capsaicin cream**
  The 0.075% cream is applied 3–4 times per day for 6 weeks.

■ **Opioids**
■ **Anticonvulsants**
  Phenytoin and carbamezepine have both been used successfully.
  More recently gabapentin has been used with some success
■ **TENS**

Reference
Grady KM, Severn AM. *Key Topics in Chronic Pain*, 1997. Bios Scientific Publishers, Oxford

Stridor post-thyroidectomy

You are called to recovery urgently to see a patient with stridor one hour following a total thyroidectomy.

What are the common causes of stridor in this situation?

■ **Wound haematoma**	Bleeding is probably the most common cause of early stridor and can lead to life-threatening respiratory obstruction. Removal of clips or sutures may help or at least buy time but tracheal intubation will be required for serious cases
■ **Bilateral RLN palsy**	Unilateral damage will cause hoarseness but bilateral damage will lead to adduction of both vocal cords and stridor
■ **Tracheal oedema**	This would be an unusual cause of stridor at such an early stage
■ **Tracheal collapse**	Tracheomalacia may occur intra- or postoperatively. It tends to occur more commonly in large or malignant goitres. A clue to its presence may be observed at the end of the operation with the absence of a leak around the cuff when it is deflated

How would you manage this situation?

This is a life-threatening scenario:

■ The patient should be given 100% oxygen
■ A consultant anaesthetist and ENT surgeon should be summoned immediately
■ If there is evidence of an expanding haematoma the skin clips should be removed although it may be necessary to open deeper layers
■ Nebulised adrenaline (5 ml of 1/1000, i.e. 5 mg) if there is a suspicion of oedema
■ Heliox (if immediately available) could be considered. **NB:** heliox is only 21% oxygen
■ The remaining causes would necessitate urgent tracheal intubation or tracheostomy

The patient deteriorates further without evidence of haematoma and requires intubation. How would you undertake this?

The anaesthetic management of this situation is contentious. The options are:

- Gas induction
- i.v. induction followed by neuromuscular blockade
- Surgical airway

Several factors may help when deciding on the most appropriate management:

- **Time.** The choice of technique will be limited by the speed of deterioration of the patient and the availability of equipment
- **Ability to achieve any ventilation.** If ventilation is not possible and the patient is becoming severely hypoxic then gas induction is clearly not an option
- **The most likely diagnosis.** The surgeon who performed the operation would know if tracheomalacia was likely – the operation note could help. Tracheomalacia may be expected to be an easier intubation than airway oedema
- **The difficulty of the original intubation**
- **Availability of a skilled ENT surgeon.** If the wound is open, there is no haematoma and the surgeon is present then a surgical airway is probably the safest option

If the patient is partially obstructed and therefore still self-ventilating, a gas induction should be performed. The patient should be immediately transferred to theatre where facilities for difficult intubation are more readily available. The patient is preoxygenated and gas induction of anaesthesia performed with sevoflurane or halothane in 100% oxygen. The trachea can then be intubated under deep inhalational anaesthesia without a muscle relaxant. The ENT surgeon should be scrubbed and ready to perform an emergency tracheostomy if oral intubation is impossible. Rigid bronchoscopy (by an experienced ENT surgeon) or transtracheal jet ventilation may be used as holding measures.

Pre-eclampsia ✓

What is the definition of pre-eclampsia?

Pre-eclampsia is a multi-system disorder occurring during pregnancy and characterised by:

- Sustained hypertension beginning after 20 weeks' gestation (systolic >140 or diastolic >90)
- Proteinuria – significant if 2+ on dipstick testing or >300 mg/24 h

It is associated with significant potential morbidity and mortality to mother and baby.

What is the underlying pathophysiology?

In normal pregnancy, there is invasion of the spiral arteries by trophoblast. They dilate and thus their resistance decreases. In pre-eclampsia, this does not occur. Instead, the **spiral arteries maintain their muscular layer and contractile ability**. This may be due to alterations in cytokine physiology. There is **placental ischaemia** and **membrane dysfunction in other organs**. Generalised vasospasm is caused by reduced prostacyclin synthesis, increased thromboxane A2 synthesis and increased sensitivity to pressors like angiotensin II.

What are the main problems associated with pre-eclampsia?

- Hypertension
- Oliguria with difficulty in assessing fluid balance and risk of pulmonary oedema
- Seizures
- Impaired coagulation
- Abnormal liver function (HELLP) and risk of hepatic rupture
- Intra-uterine growth retardation

What are the principles of management?

- Fluid balance
- Control of hypertension
- Seizure prophylaxis
- Establish epidural analgesia early if possible
- Timing and mode of delivery of the baby
- Anaesthetic techniques for delivery
- Post-delivery care

Fluid balance

Assessment of fluid balance is very difficult. There is a **contracted intra-vascular space but a tendency towards capillary leakage** and reduced colloid osmotic pressure. It is easy to give too much fluid to treat the oliguria and **pulmonary oedema is common particularly post-delivery** when interstitial fluid is mobilised. It has been shown that mothers are far more likely to die as a result of the effects of fluid overload than from renal failure secondary to hypovolaemia. Central venous pressure monitoring is only useful when the value is low to help diagnose hypovolaemia but when greater than 6 mmHg is not a reliable indicator of left ventricular filling pressure. It is important to **monitor input and output closely and avoid giving excessive volumes of fluid.** There is no difference in outcome if colloids are used instead of crystalloids.

Control of hypertension

Haemodynamic measurements tend to divide the patients into two groups. The larger, low-risk, group consists of patients with hyperdynamic left ventricular function and a moderately raised SVR. The high-risk group patients have a failing heart in association with a very high SVR. Hence, a pulmonary artery catheter (or other method of measuring CO and SVR) may be required to establish the haemodynamics and guide management. Drug therapy commonly starts with **labetolol** (7:1 β:α activity) if it is not contraindicated. **Hydralazine** may also be used, particularly in the second group, to reduce the SVR.

Epidural analgesia may also be considered as an adjunct in the management of hypertension if the platelet count and coagulation screen are OK. This is very much a risk versus benefit decision.

Seizure prophylaxis and recurrent seizures

Magnesium is probably the drug of choice. The management of seizures may be divided up into seizure prophylaxis, treatment of the first seizure and prevention of recurrent seizures.

Seizure prophylaxis

This is prevention of the first seizure. Magnesium has yet to be proved conclusively but is the subject of an on-going trial. It is, however, the most commonly used drug in this context.

Treatment of acute seizures

May be undertaken with drugs such as magnesium, diazepam or thiopentone. Magnesium is now the most commonly used drug for this purpose and is recommended in a dose of 2 g if already on a magnesium infusion.

Prevention of recurrent seizures

The efficacy of magnesium is now well established and it should be the first-line therapy (**Collaborative Eclampsia Trial** showed it to be clearly superior to phenytoin and diazepam).

Magnesium therapy:

- **Dose = 4 g bolus** over 10 minutes followed by an infusion of 1–2 g/h
- **Therapeutic level = 2–3.5 mmol/L**
- **Continue for 24 hours after last seizure**
- **Magnesium 1g = 4 mmol**

Symptoms and signs of hypermagnesaemia:

- Nausea and flushing
- Somnolence
- Double vision
- Slurred speech
- ↓ **patellar reflexes – first sign**   > 5 mmol/L
- Respiratory depression   > 6 mmol/L
- Respiratory arrest   6.3–7.1 mmol/L
- Cardiac arrest at   12.5–14.6 mmol/L

Magnesium may work by prevention of cerebral vasospasm through the block of Ca^{2+} influx via NMDA glutamate channels.

Establish epidural analgesia

If timing and the clinical state of the patient permit then siting an epidural under controlled conditions is ideal. If a caesarian section is required later and the **epidural** has already been sited then it can be topped-up for theatre. Coagulation tests and platelet count need to be checked prior to the procedure.

Timing and mode of delivery

This needs to be decided by the obstetrician and anaesthetist in collaboration and will be determined by the clinical situation.

Anaesthetic techniques for delivery

If an urgent caesarian section is required and there is no time to establish an epidural then the choice is limited to spinal or general anaesthesia. **Spinal anaesthesia** remains controversial because of the risk of hypotension and uteroplacental insufficiency although there have been several publications in the recent literature describing its use. If a regional block is contra-indicated, for example because of coagulopathy, or there is no time because of severe foetal distress then **general anaesthesia** will have to be undertaken. Factors making GA in pre-eclampsia particularly hazardous include a higher chance of difficult intubation and a marked pressor response at laryngoscopy and intubation. There is a significant risk of intracerebral haemorrhage secondary to severe hypertension. Invasive monitoring should be established pre-induction if there is time.

Post-delivery care

Convulsions can occur up to 23 days after delivery. In the UK up to 44% of fits occur in the puerperium. Fluid balance can remain difficult in the postoperative period. The most common time for pulmonary oedema to occur is in the first 48–72 hours post-delivery. This is probably a result of large volumes of fluid given peri-operatively (in the face of oliguria and capillary-leak syndrome) mobilising from the extravascular space as the patient improves. Platelet count is lowest in the 24–48 hours post-delivery and HELLP presents after delivery in 30% of cases. This demonstrates that although delivery of the baby is the 'cure', it may not be the end of the problem. The decision to send a patient to **intensive care** is made on the basis of her clinical condition (a patient may also be considered for intensive care pre-operatively).

References

Brodie H, Malinow AM. Anaesthetic management of pre-eclampsia/eclampsia. Review article, *IJOA*, April 1999

Engelhardt T, Maclennan FM. Fluid management in pre-eclampsia. Review article, *IJOA*, October 1999

Mortl MG, Schneider MC. Key issues in assessing, managing and treating patients presenting with severe pre-eclampsia. Review article, *IJOA*, January 2000

Premedication

What are the indications for premedication in modern anaesthetic practice?

This question can be answered in a list fashion in the knowledge that the examiner will want you to elaborate on a number of your answers. The main indications are as follows:

Think of the seven A's

- Anxiolysis
- Amnesia
- Antiemesis
- Analgesia – systemic and topical (for venepuncture)
- Antacids
- Antisialogogues
- Additional – oxygen, nebulisers, steroids, heparin, etc.

Tell me what you would use for:

'Anxiolysis/Amnesia'

It is worth mentioning that the **preoperative visit** is an important component of anxiolysis by establishing a rapport with the patient, discussing the anaesthetic technique and answering any questions they may have. Parental anxiety can also be addressed at this stage.

- **Benzodiazepines** are probably the most commonly prescribed premedicants. They act by enhancing GABA, an inhibitory neurotransmitter that causes an influx of chloride ions thereby hyperpolarising the neurone. They produce anxiolysis, amnesia and sedation and can be given orally, intramuscularly or intranasally. Typical doses are:

Temazepam	10–30 mg orally in adults
	0.5–1 mg/kg orally in children upto 20 mg
Midazolam	0.2–0.75 mg/kg orally in children (max 20 mg)
	5–10 mg i.m.
	0.2–0.3 mg/kg intranasally
Lorazepam	2–4 mg orally
Diazepam	5–10 mg orally in adults
	0.2–0.4 mg/kg orally in children

- **Trimeprazine** (2 mg/kg), a phenothiazine with anticholinergic, antihistamine, antidopaminergic and α-blocking properties is used less commonly
- The newer α_2–**agonists** clonidine and dexmedetomidine reduce sympathetic outflow and have been used as premedicants, with sedative, anxiolytic and analgesic properties.

'Antiemesis'

Most anaesthetists would target specific groups of patients at high risk of postoperative nausea and vomiting for preoperative antiemetics:

- Previous history of PONV/motion sickness (3× incidence of PONV)
- Those having 'high-risk' surgery, e.g. gynaecological, upper abdominal, middle ear and squint surgery.
- Females (2–4× that of males)
- Obese patients
- Other risk factors – use of opiates, nitrous oxide, volatile versus TIVA

The choice of antiemetics is then from 5–HT$_3$, dopamine, histamine or muscarinic antagonists.

- Dopamine antagonists: This group includes the phenothiazines (commonly prochlorperazine), butyrophenones (droperidol) and metoclopramide. The evidence for the efficacy of these drugs is often variable and they can produce extra-pyramidal side-effects, e.g. dyskinesia, tremor, dystonia and oculogyric crisis.
- Histamine antagonists: These act directly on the vomiting centre, e.g. cyclizine
- Muscarinic antagonists: This group, which includes hyoscine and atropine, is probably used less commonly than in times when reducing excessive secretions was an important component of premedication. Side-effects include dry mouth, blurred vision, sedation and disorientation in elderly patients.
- 5HT$_3$ antagonists: The advantage of these drugs, e.g. ondansetron, is their efficacy and side-effect profile compared to the more traditional agents. They are, however, more expensive.

Other modalities include:

- Dexamethasone
- Acupuncture and acupressure
- NK$_1$ antagonists
- Cannabinoids

Some evidence is coming through that combination therapy may be more useful than single agent prophylaxis but the optimal timing of administering these agents has yet to be established.

'Analgesia'

Routine opioid premedication for elective surgery is used less frequently than in years gone by and the concept of pre-emptive analgesia (modulating spinal cord nociceptive transmission) has yet to be translated into a proven clinical entity. Treating acute preoperative pain should be guided by the clinical situation.

In paediatric practice, EMLA™ cream is commonly used as a topical anaesthetic before venepuncture. This is the Eutectic Mixture of Local

Anaesthetics and is a mixture of the unionised forms of lignocaine and prilocaine. It should be applied for at least 1 hour with an occlusive dressing covering it.

'Antacids'

The overall incidence of aspiration related to anaesthesia has been quoted as 1:3216, with a higher incidence for emergency surgery (1:895). Of these, 64% do not develop any further symptoms and 20% require mechanical ventilation. It is interesting to note that Warner *et al* found no difference in the aspiration rate if pharmacoprophylaxis was used or not.

There are many risk factors that have been associated with perioperative aspiration, e.g. emergency surgery, obstetrics, obesity and hiatus hernia. Historically, a significant residual volume of gastric juice (>0.4 ml/kg) and low pH (below 2.5) were thought to be important factors. This has since been questioned.

The main drugs used to alter gastric secretions are:

- H_2-antagonists – these agents e.g. ranitidine alter both the production and pH of gastric contents.
- Sodium citrate is used to neutralise the pH of gastric contents, particularly in the obstetric setting
- Prokinetic agents such as metoclopramide

References

Ahmed AB *et al*. Randomised, placebo-controlled trial of combination antiemetic prophylaxis for day-case gynaecological laparoscopic surgery. *BJA*, 2000, Volume 85(5), p678–682

Warner MA, Warner ME, Weber JG. Clinical significance of pulmonary aspiration during the perioperative period. *Anaesthesiology*, 1993, Volume 78, p56–62

Raised intracranial pressure therapy

When treating a patient with a severe head injury on the intensive care unit we talk about using cerebral protection.

What does this mean?

Cerebral protection means controlling the physiological and biochemical milieu of the brain to **decrease the likelihood of secondary brain injury**.

Several factors have been shown to be associated with poor outcome after severe head injury. These are:

- Increasing age
- Low admission GCS
- Pupillary signs
- Systolic blood pressure <90 mmHg
- Low arterial O_2 tension
- High arterial CO_2 tension
- ICP >20 mmHg
- High blood glucose

Attention must therefore be paid to controlling these factors. An adequate cerebral perfusion pressure (some suggest >70 mmHg or until pressure waves disappear from the ICP waveform) must be maintained and hypoxia should be avoided at all costs. A 'low–normal' $PaCO_2$ (35–40 mmHg) is current best practice. Any patient with a severe head injury should have their ICP monitored and should preferably be cared for in a neurosurgical intensive care unit.

What are the causes of primary cerebral injury?

This is the damage that occurs at the time of the initial insult and may be the result of:

- Trauma
- Haemorrhage
- Tumour

What is secondary brain injury?

This is additional ischaemic neurological damage that occurs after the initial injury as a result of:

- Hypoxaemia
- Hypercapnia
- Hypotension
- Raised ICP
- Cerebral arterial spasm

Possible mechanisms

Glutamate and aspartate act on NMDA receptors causing increased intracellular calcium, activation of phospholipases, breakdown of arachidonic acid and generation of free radicals.

What CO_2 do we aim for and why?

At a $PaCO_2$ between 3.0 kPa (23 mmHg) and 7.0 kPa (53 mmHg) cerebral blood flow is directly proportional to the $PaCO_2$. In the past hyperventilation has been used to decrease CBF and CBV, but it has been shown that **hyperventilation (CO_2 less than 35mmHg) is associated with a poorer outcome** because it may produce ischaemia secondary to a severe reduction in CBF. A **'low–normal' CO_2 of just over 4.6 kPa (35 mmHg)** is now the accepted target.

How can we treat raised ICP?

Treatment of raised ICP should be initiated if >20–25 mmHg and is aimed at reducing the volume of the three components making up the intracranial contents: namely brain, blood and CSF. Firstly, **maintenance of an adequate cerebral perfusion pressure** should be ensured. Arterial blood gases should be corrected. The patient should be sedated to a satisfactory level. Attention can then be paid to the following:

Decreasing the brain volume
- Mannitol (0.25–1.0 g/kg) is frequently used to reduce cerebral oedema.
- Loop diuretics e.g. frusemide (0.5 mg/kg) given within 10–15 min of mannitol produce a synergistic effect. They encourage a more hypotonic diuresis that prolongs the duration of intravascular osmotic load produced by mannitol
- Cerebral oedema may be worsened with inattention to the serum osmolarity, which should be kept between 300 and 310 mosmol. Hypotonic solutions should be avoided. Treat diabetes insipidus with DDAVP
- Surgical removal of brain tissue

Decreasing cerebral blood volume (CBV)
- Surgical removal of blood (i.e. clot)
- Avoid impeding venous drainage by tight tube ties, high ventilation pressures or excessive neck rotation
- Venous drainage can be aided by a 30° head-up position
- Hyperventilation can be effective in the short term but should not be used in the long term because of the potential for causing ischaemia (can be monitored by jugular bulb venous oxygen saturation and cerebral oximetry)
- Reducing cerebral metabolic requirements with thiopentone will decrease cerebral blood volume by decreasing cerebral blood flow, but has the disadvantage of prolonged sedation
- Control of fitting (fitting increases $CMRO_2$ and therefore cerebral blood flow)
- Avoidance of pyrexia will help to prevent increases in the $CMRO_2$ and associated increases in CBF and ICP. Induced hypothermia has been used in an attempt to improve outcome. However, a recent multicentre study does not support its routine use

Head injury and hypothermia

A study published in the *New England Journal of Medicine* (Feb 2001) looked at the effect of induced hypothermia (to 33°C) on outcome at 6 months after closed head injury. The trial was stopped after 392 patients (500 planned) because there was no improvement in outcome and in fact patients in the over-45-years group did worse. The authors recommended not deliberately cooling patients who were normothermic on admission. However, if they were hypothermic on admission then they should not be aggressively warmed.

Decreasing the CSF volume
- CSF can be drained via an external ventricular drain (EVD)
- Production is reduced by mannitol and frusemide

Mannitol

- Osmotic diuretic
- Rheological effects   ↓ red cell rigidity (rbc membrane)
  ↓ haematocrit (haemodilution)
- Free-radical scavenger
- Dose is usually 0.5 g/kg rapid infusion
- Giving frusemide 0.5 mg/kg 10–15 minutes after mannitol prolongs its effect (see above)
- Efficacy depends on intact BBB

References
Clifton GL *et al.* Lack of effect of induction of hypothermia after acute brain injury. *New England Journal of Medicine,* February 2001, Volume 344(8), p556–563
Galley HF. *Critical Care Focus 3: Neurological Injury.* BMJ Books
Kaufmann. *Anaesthesia Review 13.* Churchill Livingstone, Edinburgh
The management of raised intracranial pressure. CME Core Topic. *BJA Bulletin* 1 May 2000
Stone DJ *et al. The Neuroanaesthesia Handbook,* 1996. Mosby, St Louis, Missouri, USA

Rheumatoid arthritis

What are the clinical features of rheumatoid arthritis?

This is a chronic multisystem autoimmune disease of unknown cause. It principally affects the joints causing a **symmetrical inflammatory polyarthritis**. This presents as **pain and stiffness**. Most patients have several joints involved, especially the hands, wrists, elbows, shoulders, cervical spine, knees, ankles and feet.

Other findings are **Sjögren's syndrome** (dry eyes and dry mouth), **Felty's syndrome** (splenomegaly and neutropenia), **anaemia** and **thrombocytopenia**.

Other systems involved include:

■ **The respiratory system**	Pleural effusions
	Diffuse fibrosing alveolitis
	Nodules
	Caplan's syndrome
	Small airways disease
■ **The cardiovascular system**	Up to 35% of patients
	Pericarditis
	Nodules causing conduction defects
	Tamponade – rarely
	Endocarditis (usually mitral)
■ **The haemopoietic system**	Anaemia (see later)
	Effects of drug treatment
■ **The kidneys**	40% have impaired renal function
	Amyloidosis
	Drug toxicity
■ **The skin**	Leg ulcers
	Vasculitic lesions
■ **The CNS**	Polyneuropathy
	Carpal tunnel syndrome
	Atlanto-axial subluxation

What airway problems can rheumatoid arthritis present?

■ **Cervical instability** caused by weakening of the transverse ligament of the atlas resulting in potential cord compression. Assess with flexion and extension X-rays looking for a 3 mm gap between odontoid peg and posterior border of anterior arch of atlas
■ **Limited cervical spine movement**
■ **Fixed flexion deformity** is not uncommon
■ **Cricoarytenoid involvement** can result in upper airway obstruction (hoarseness and stridor)
■ **Temporomandibular joint** involvement may limit mouth opening

A **difficult intubation** is therefore likely and consideration should be given to spinal/epidural anaesthesia or a LMA technique. Otherwise an awake fibreoptic intubation may be necessary.

What are the <u>other</u> problems associated with anaesthesia in these patients?

These are:

■ **Respiratory problems**
A restrictive lung defect may be present and will warrant investigation with pre-op pulmonary function tests, a chest X-ray and blood gases

■ **Anaemia**
Anaemia of chronic disease (normochromic, normocytic)
Iron deficiency – GI bleeding from use of NSAIDs
Bone marrow suppression from gold and penicillamine
Haemolytic anaemia
Felty's syndrome causing hypersplenism
■ **Other systemic complications** of the disease, e.g. CVS/renal problems
■ **Positioning**
Care is required due to fixed deformities, tendon and muscle contractures
and fragile skin (long-term steroid therapy). Access for local anaesthetic
techniques may be difficult
■ **Monitoring**
Inserting invasive monitoring lines can be very difficult for the same
reasons
■ **Altered response to drugs**
Renal dysfunction
Decreased serum albumin
Increased α_1–acid glycoprotein
■ **Concomitant drug therapy**
■ **Postoperatively**
May be unable to use a PCA

What are the complications of drug therapy?

Commonly prescribed medication includes:

■ **NSAIDs**	Renal impairment, gastric erosions, bleeding
	Fluid retention
■ **Steroids**	Hypertension, electrolyte imbalance, diabetes
	Easy bruising, osteoporosis, obesity, myopathy, mania
	Peptic ulcer disease, etc.
■ **Penicillamine**	Bone marrow suppression (thrombocytopenia, neutropenia, agranulocytosis)
	Haemolytic anaemia
	Nephrotic syndrome
	SLE-like syndrome
	Myasthenia-like syndrome
■ **Chloroquine**	Retinopathy
	Cardiomyopathy
■ **Gold**	Fatal blood disorders
	Pulmonary fibrosis
	Hepatotoxicity
	Nephrotic syndrome
■ **Azathioprine**	Bone marrow suppression
	Abnormal LFTs
■ **Methotrexate**	Pulmonary toxicity (esp. in rheumatoid patients)
	Cirrhosis
	Blood dyscrasias

■ **Sulphasalazine**   GI side effects
Haematological toxicity
■ **Cyclosporin**   Nephrotoxicity

Reference

Skues MA, Welchew EA. Anaesthesia and rheumatoid arthritis. *Anaesthesia* 1993, Volume 48, p989–997

Sickle cell

An unbooked Afro-Caribbean primigravida arrives on the ward in advanced labour. Fetal distress is diagnosed and the obstetricians wish to do an emergency caesarean section. Her full blood count shows an Hb of 8.3 g/dl with a microcytic picture (normal platelets). Time will not permit electrophoresis.

What may explain the blood picture?

A haemoglobin concentration of less than 10.5 g/dl is due to something other than the dilutional anaemia of pregnancy. Some causes of a microcytic anaemia with normal platelets are:

- Iron deficiency
- Hb SS (Sickle cell disease) – the patient would know this diagnosis
- **Hb AS** (Sickle cell trait)
- **Hb SC**
- α-Thalassaemia
- β-Thalassaemia (less common in Africans)
- Some anaemias of chronic disease

The blood film should be examined and electrophoresis should be organised because it may influence future management.

Sickle cell trait (AS)
- Usually no clinical abnormality unless exposed to extreme hypoxia (sickling if $PaO_2 < 15$ mmHg)
- Increased risk of pyelonephritis during pregnancy

Sickle cell-haemoglobin C (SC) disease
- Less severe clinical course than SCD but can suffer the same complications
- Prevalent in West Africans
- May not develop symptoms until late pregnancy (splenic sequestration and marrow necrosis)
- Can develop proliferative retinopathy

How would you manage anaesthesia for the caesarean section?

Pregnancy exacerbates the complications of sickle cell anaemia. Maternal mortality of 1% is due to pulmonary infection and infarction.
Blood transfusions are indicated for:

- Severe anaemia
- Hypoxemia
- Pre-eclampsia
- Septicaemia
- Renal failure
- Acute chest pain syndrome
- Anticipated surgery

A haemoglobin concentration of 10 g/dL is commonly aimed for in patients having a caesarean section.

Either regional or general anaesthesia is acceptable. Principles of management are:

- Oxygen
- Crystalloids for intravascular volume
- Transfusion to maintain oxygen-carrying capacity
- Venous stasis prophylaxis
- Normothermia

Anaesthetic problems with sickle cell disease:

- Avoidance of precipitants of sickle crises
- Difficult i.v. access
- Pain/opioid tolerance
- Anaemia and high output failure
- Infection (salmonella)
- Psychiatric problems
- Intra-operative crisis/thrombo-embolic phenomena
- Acute chest syndrome
- Renal impairment
- Pulmonary hypertension

Precipitants of a sickle crisis:

- Dehydration
- Hypoxia
- Cold
- Alcohol
- Stress
- Infection
- Menstruation
- Vascular stasis
- Acidosis

Surgery proceeds uneventfully but postoperatively she develops acute pleuritic chest pain. What may be causing this?

Possible causes
- Pulmonary embolus
- Acute chest syndrome
- Pneumothorax
- Pneumonia

If this were a sickle crisis, how would you manage the case?

The mainstays of management of a sickle crisis are:

- Analgesia
- Fluid replacement
- Avoidance of hypoxia

Types of sickle crisis:

- **Aplastic**   Depression of erythropoiesis secondary to infection (esp. parvovirus) or folate deficiency in pregnancy
- **Sequestration**   This can result from massive pooling in the spleen (esp. with SC disease)
- **Infarctive**   These are vaso-occlusive events, often in the abdomen, back or long bones

---

- **Pain**   Can be very severe (and often underestimated)

  Treat with: High-dose opioids (PCA may be used)

      NSAIDs

      Epidural

      Paracetamol

      Fentanyl patches

      Tricyclic antidepressants

      Benzodiazepines for spasms and anxiolysis

- **Dehydration** causes increased haematocrit and increased sickling

- If **fever** is present: Search for focus of infection (**cultures** of blood, sputum and urine)

  It may be due to the **crisis itself**

  Broad-spectrum antibiotics, which must cover *Strep. pneumonii* (hyposplenism)

- If refractory: **Exchange transfusion**

  Steroids have been used (Methylprednisolone)

Acute Chest Syndrome

Cause   Unknown exactly

    ? Hypoventilation due to pain from rib infarcts

    ? infarcted marrow embolism

    ? PE

Signs   Acute chest pain

    Fever

    Cough

    Basal X-ray changes

    $\downarrow SaO_2$

Treatment O_2/CPAP/IPPV

    Exchange transfusion with HbS < 30% causes a response within 1–2 days

Sickling mechanism

The HbS tetramer undergoes a conformational change in the **deoxygenated** state and leaves **hydrophobic residues** (valine instead of glutamic acid) exposed. These react with other globin chains forming an **insoluble polymer**. HbS begins to aggregate at a PO_2 of less than 50 mmHg. The process is also time dependent.

When exposed to **oxidant stress**, HbS produces **free radicals** that damage the erythrocyte membrane proteins. **Abnormal adhesion to endothelium** then occurs.

Infection or minor sickling events cause leucocytes to produce **IL-6, IL-1 and TNF** that **upregulate cell adhesion molecules** (CAMs) on the vascular endothelium. These cause **activation of the haemostatic mechanism**. Platelets and sickle reticulocytes bind easily to CAMs causing **clot formation and vascular occlusion** → **hypoxia** → more sickling.

References

Chestnut DH. *Obstetric Anesthesia: Principles and Practice*, 1994. Mosby, St Louis, USA

Esseltine DW, Baxter MRN, Bevan JC. Sickle cell states and the anaesthetist. *Canadian Journal of Anaesthesia*, July 1988, Volume 35(4), p385–403

Hatton C, Mackie PH. Haemoglobinopathies and other congenital haemolytic anaemias. *Medicine*, January 1996, Volume 24(1), p14–19

Hoffbrand AV, Pettit JE. *Essential Haematology*, third edition, 1993. Blackwell Scientific Publications, Oxford, UK

Vijay V, Cavenagh JD, Yate P. The anaesthetist's role in acute sickle cell crisis. *BJA*, June 1998, Volume 80, p820–828

Tension pneumothorax

A 35-year-old man has sustained a fall from a ladder and presents to the accident department with increasing shortness of breath.

What does his CXR show?

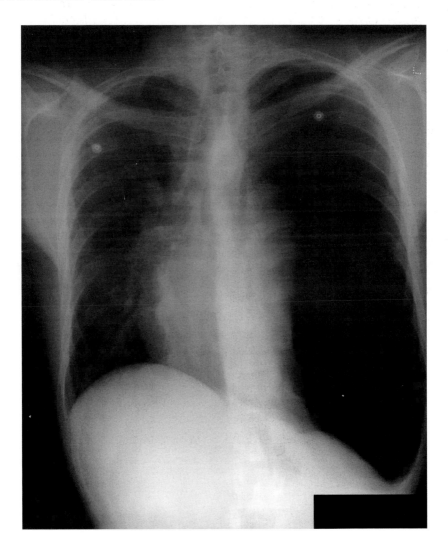

This is a left tension pneumothorax. There is gross mediastinal shift to the right. This needs immediate treatment.

How would you treat this?

- Administer high-flow oxygen
- Identify the 2nd intercostal space in the midclavicular line on the side of the pneumothorax

- Surgically prepare the chest and locally anaesthetise the area if time permits
- Insert a cannula (14 or 16 gauge) into the space passing just superior to the rib and puncturing the parietal pleura to enter the pleural cavity
- Remove the needle and listen for a rush of air to confirm placement and diagnosis
- Insert a definitive chest drain and remove the original cannula
- Obtain a chest X-ray

What are the complications of this procedure?

- Pneumothorax
- Local bleeding (intercostal vessel damage)
- Local cellulitis
- Pleural infection

Reference
Advanced Trauma Life Support Course for Physicians. American College of Surgeons, 1993

Tetanus

A 47-year-old farmer presents with dysphagia, malaise and muscle pains following a minor accident at work 6 days earlier.

Tell me some causes of dysphagia.

It is important to have some form of sieve for an answer like this that you may not have directly thought about before. You will know most of the causes, but delivering them in a structured format will look slick.

Mechanical	Benign internal stricture, e.g. oesophageal web
	Malignant internal stricture, e.g. oesophageal/gastric cancer
	Extrinsic pressure, e.g. lung cancer, retrosternal goitre
	Pharyngeal pouch
Motility problems	Bulbar palsy
	Pseudobulbar palsy
	Achalasia
	Systemic sclerosis
	Myasthenia gravis
	Rare infective causes, e.g. tetanus, Chagas' disease
Others	Oesophagitis

What is the likely diagnosis in this farmer?

The most likely diagnosis from the history is tetanus.

What is the causative organism?

The disease is caused by **exotoxins produced by *Clostridium tetani***, an obligate anaerobic, spore-bearing, Gram-positive bacillus. The spores exist in the soil and gastrointestinal tract of humans and animals. The organism is non-invasive but the spores can gain entry through wounds, ulcers, etc. where they can proliferate and produce the toxins **tetanospasmin** (an extremely potent protein) and tetanolysin. Tetanospasmin is taken up and transmitted by neural pathways to the central nervous system where it **preferentially binds to inhibitory interneurones** thereby blocking these pathways and allowing uninhibited afferent stimuli.

   C. tetani is difficult to culture and only identified in about one third of cases.

What is the natural course of the disease?

The incubation period is from 1 day to several months. There is a prodrome of non-specific stiffness, fever, malaise, headache and dysphagia. This is followed by the classical symptoms of:

- Trismus   'Lockjaw' due to masseter spasm
- Risus sardonicus   Rigidity and spasm in the facial muscles
- Opisthotonus   Arched body secondary to paravertebral muscle spasm
- Painful spasms may eventually compromise respiration
- Sympathetic overactivity   Tachycardia, arrhythmias, paroxysmal hypertension, sweating, pyrexia and gastrointestinal stasis.

The spasms can be precipitated by noise, handling or even light.

How would you treat this man?

- In the first instance an ABC approach is adopted and further management guided by clinical findings
- The wound should be cleaned and debrided
- Give benzylpenicillin
- To neutralise the free toxin, human tetanus immunoglobulin is given i.m.
- General nursing care is very important. These patients should be nursed in a quiet, isolated, darkened room
- Diazepam or chlorpromazine should be given initially to try and control the spasms
- Dantrolene has been used in the treatment of tetanic spasms
- Magnesium may also be used to control spasms
- Intensive care may be indicated with paralysis and ventilation
- Ventilation is likely to be prolonged if required and early tracheostomy should be considered

- Autonomic dysfunction often occurs after the onset of respiratory symptoms and can be treated with β-blockers, e.g. labetolol
- Other general ICU measures include nutritional support and thromboprophylaxis
- Mortality, even with supportive intensive care, is around 11%
- Patients die from aspiration, hypoxia, respiratory failure and cardiac arrest

References

Craft TM, Upton PM. *Key Topics in Anaesthesia*, 2nd edition. Bios Scientific Publishers, 1995, Oxford
Hinds CJ, Watson D. *Intensive Care. A concise textbook*, 2nd edition, 1996. Baillière Tindall, London

Thyroidectomy

What are the anaesthetic problems of a patient who is thyrotoxic with a large goitre presenting for thyroidectomy?

These may be divided into the effects of thyrotoxicosis and those of the goitre on the airway and surrounding structures.

Thyrotoxicosis

■ Cardiovascular	Tachycardia
	Arrhythmias (esp. AF)
	Congestive cardiac failure
	Ischaemic heart disease
	May be chronically hypovolaemic and vasodilated causing hypotension on induction
	Exaggerated response to laryngoscopy and surgical stimulation with tachycardia, hypertension and ventricular arrhythmias
■ Thyroid storm	See below
■ Eyes	Lid retraction, exophthalmos, conjunctivitis
■ Other	Proximal myopathy
	Anaemia
	Thrombocytopenia
	Hypercalcaemia
	Abnormal glucose tolerance
	Associated auto-immune disease – e.g. diabetes, myasthenia

Effects of goitre

■ Compression	
Airway	May be worse in supine position, eased on side or prone
	Tracheomalacia (especially postoperatively)
SVC	Retrosternal extension
	Oedematous face and airway

Engorgement of nasopharyngeal veins (epistaxis with fibreoptic intubation)

Poor venous return therefore place i.v. line in lower extremity (IVC territory)

Recurrent laryngeal nerve

1% have involvement preoperatively. This causes cord adduction leading to a hoarse voice.

Bilateral nerve involvement causes stridor.

- **Tumour invasion of local tissues**

How would you assess her thyroid status?

Symptoms	Weight loss, diarrhoea, vomiting
	Restlessness, tremor
	Palpitations
	Heat intolerance
	Eye complications (Graves' disease)
Signs	Tachycardia
	Atrial fibrillation
	Cardiac failure
	Warm, vasodilated peripheries
	Goitre with bruit
	Hyperkinesis
Investigations	TSH ↓
	T3 ↑
	T4 ↑
	Free T4 ↑
	Thyroid scan (^{131}I) – 'hot' or 'cold' spots

Which drugs are used to manage thyrotoxicosis?

Carbimazole	Inhibits hormone synthesis
	Takes 4–8 weeks to work
	Major side effect is depression of the white cell count
	Agranulocytosis in 1/1000 after 3 months
Propylthiouracil	Inhibits hormone synthesis
	Also inhibits peripheral conversion of T4 to more active T3
	Given if sensitive to carbimazole
	Takes 4–8 weeks to work
	Side-effects include leucopenia, aplastic anaemia, lupus-like syndrome
Iodine	(Lugol's solution) Traditionally given for 10 days prior to surgery to reduce the vascularity of the gland. This practice is now less common because the thyroid gland is dissected without transection

■ **β-blocker**　　　　　Propranolol controls cardiovascular effects and decreases peripheral conversion of T4 to more active T3
Heart rate of less than 85 has been recommended
Atenolol or nadolol (both longer acting) may achieve better control of symptoms

How would you assess the airway?

■ **Symptoms**　　　　Positional dyspnoea (esp. supine with retrosternal goitre)
Dysphagia

■ **Signs**　　　　　　Stridor
Routine assessment of expected difficulty with intubation

■ **Investigations**　　Indirect laryngoscopy or fibreoptic nasendoscopy by ENT surgeon will give clues as to whether the larynx is likely to be easily visualised at direct laryngoscopy
Chest X-ray/lateral thoracic inlet – tracheal compression/deviation
CT scan – extension of retrosternal goitre and site/degree of tracheal compression. Diameter of airway at narrowest point can also be measured

If we postulate that this patient was euthyroid with no clinical or radiological evidence of obstruction, how would you anaesthetise her?

■ Premedication　　Benzodiazepine
β-blocker continued

■ Standard i.v. induction and muscle relaxation is acceptable
■ Care to obtund pressor responses
■ Armoured tube – well-secured
■ Attention to eye protection
■ Sandbag between shoulder blades
■ Head up (reduces bleeding) and extended
■ Arms by the side therefore long drip extensions
■ Check cords at the end when breathing spontaneously – bilateral recurrent laryngeal nerve damage will cause bilateral cord adduction and stridor
■ Extubate 'awake'
■ Post-operative care to include attention to oxygenation, fluid balance, analgesia, airway monitoring for signs of obstruction – clip remover immediately available
■ Check serum calcium and have i.v. calcium by the bedside
■ Continue β-blocker

What is thyroid storm and how is it managed?

This is a life-threatening syndrome seen in hyperthyroid patients typically 6–24 hours postoperatively although it may occur intra-operatively. It is characterised by hyperpyrexia, tachycardia, hypotension and altered consciousness. It may initially mimic malignant hyperthermia but is not associated with muscle rigidity or a rise in CK. Other factors such as labour or severe infection may also precipitate the syndrome.

Treatment consists of:

■ Antithyroid drugs   Propylthiouracil – orally or N/G
                      Iodide – inhibits release of hormone from gland
                      Dexamethasone – inhibits synthesis, release and peripheral conversion
■ β-blocker   Propranolol – combined β_1 and β_2 preferable
                      β_1 Cardiovascular effects
                      β_2 Suppresses metabolic effects
                      Reduces muscle blood flow and therefore heat production
■ Active cooling
■ i.v. fluids
■ Paracetamol
■ Invasive monitoring and inotropic/vasopressor therapy as indicated

References

Craft T, Upton P. *Key Topics in Anaesthesia*, 1995. Bios Scientific Publishers, Oxford
Deakin CD. *Clinical Notes for the FRCA*, 1998. Churchill Livingstone, Edinburgh
Farling PA. Thyroid disease. *BJA*, 2000, Volume 85(1), p15–28
Goldstone J, Pollard B. *Handbook of Clinical Anaesthesia* 1996. Churchill Livingstone, Edinburgh
Hagberg CA. *Handbook of Difficult Airway Management*, 2000. Churchill Livingstone, Philadelphia, USA
Kumar P, Clark M. *Clinical Medicine*, 1994. Baillière Tindall, London
Morgan GE, Mikhail MS. *Clinical Anaesthesiology*, 2nd edition, 1996. Appleton and Lange, Stamford, CT

Trauma

You are called to casualty to assess a 25-year-old male pedestrian who has been hit by a car at unknown speed. He was unconscious at the scene and has an obvious compound fracture of his right tibia and fibula. His foot is cool and dusky. He is agitated and his GCS is now 14. The orthopaedic surgeons want to fix his leg as soon as possible.

How would you assess this patient?

This is a **major trauma** case and he should be **assessed** and **resuscitated** according to the **ATLS guidelines**. From the history he could have sustained occult life-threatening injuries such as a fractured pelvis, intra-abdominal or intra-cerebral haemorrhage.

T

Assessment
■ **Airway and cervical spine**
   Look for evidence of airway obstruction, especially facial fractures and
   foreign bodies in the mouth
■ **Breathing**
   Expose the chest and examine for adequacy of ventilation: Inspection,
   palpation, percussion, auscultation
   Measure SaO_2 and respiratory rate

> **Beware at this point:**
>
> ■ **Tension pneumothorax**
> ■ **Flail chest**
> ■ **Open pneumothorax**
> ■ **Massive haemothorax**

■ **Circulation**
   Skin colour and capillary refill
   Pulse, ECG
   Blood pressure
   Level of consciousness
   This patient is likely to have sustained a head injury. It is therefore vital
   to maintain mean arterial pressure in order to optimise cerebral
   perfusion pressure
■ **Dysfunction**
   AVPU
   GCS
■ **Exposure**
   To complete the primary survey

After a thorough assessment of his injuries in casualty it is important to
prioritise his further management, e.g. potential life-threatening
haemorrhage from his abdomen takes precedence over a potential head
injury.

What investigations would you like before taking him to theatre?

■ Cervical spine, chest and pelvis X-rays
■ Haemoglobin and cross-match, urea, electrolytes and glucose
■ If there is any cardiovascular instability with no obvious cause or there are
   positive abdominal signs then further investigation of the abdomen is
   indicated. This may take the form of diagnostic peritoneal lavage,
   ultrasound or CT scan. A general surgeon should be present from the
   outset as part of the trauma team
■ In view of the history a CT scan of his head is indicated to exclude
   intracranial pathology such as haemorrhage or oedema

The patient is too agitated to tolerate a CT scan. How would you manage this situation?

This patient now requires a general anaesthetic for his CT scan. He also needs an anaesthetic for his tibia and fibula fracture. Although a regional technique would be ideal for his lower limb surgery it is not practical because of his agitation. A central neuroaxial block may also have detrimental effects on cerebral blood flow due to the fall in mean arterial pressure. In addition to this, there is the theoretical risk of coning associated with dural puncture.

He could be anaesthetised in casualty with a rapid sequence induction and intubation with C-spine immobilisation (either by hard collar or Manual In-Line Stabilisation). It is important to pay careful attention to measures that help prevent a rise in intracranial pressure.

If there is vascular compromise in the leg then manipulation and temporary stabilisation could be performed after the patient has been anaesthetised and is being prepared for transfer to the CT scanner.

Reference
Advanced Trauma Life Support Course for Physicians. American College of Surgeons, 1993

Trigeminal neuralgia

What are the clinical features of a patient with trigeminal neuralgia?

Recurrent, short-lived, paroxysms of sudden onset and severe, lancinating pain in the distribution of one or more branches of the trigeminal nerve. The most common sites are the mandibular branch alone followed by maxillary followed by both together. The pain is usually unilateral but may be bilateral in 3–5% of cases. The patient typically has a trigger zone.

What is the differential diagnosis?

■ **'Primary'** trigeminal neuralgia (80% of cases) is caused by an abnormal vascular loop (usually arterial) at the **dorsal root entry zone** in the apex of the petrous temporal bone (trigeminal cave). It is present in about 60% of primary cases. This compresses the nerve resulting in the characteristic clinical features. It may be detected by Magnetic Resonance Imaging
■ **Postherpetic neuralgia**
■ **Lesions by site:**
  Brainstem   Tumour
                           Multiple sclerosis (18% of bilateral cases have MS)
                           Infarct
                           Syringobulbia

T

Cerebellopontine angle	Acoustic neuroma
	Meningioma
Apex of petrous temporal bone	Middle ear infection
Cavernous sinus	ICA aneurysm
	Tumour
	Cavernous sinus thrombosis

What features suggest primary trigeminal neuralgia?

- **Asymptomatic between attacks.** Patients with another aetiology as listed above may complain of persistent pain.
- **Absence of neurological signs.** The presence of *any* neurological signs suggests a secondary cause and should be investigated as such.

What treatment options are available?

Treatment will be determined by the cause and the suitability for surgery.

- **Surgical** — **Microvascular decompression** (MVD) involves craniotomy and the associated anaesthetic and surgical risks. If an artery is found to be the cause of the compression it is dissected away and held clear of the nerve. Veins may be ligated. 'Minor' surgical interventions include radiofrequency rhizolysis and glycerol rhizolysis
- **Pharmacological** — Usually involves the use of anticonvulsants such as carbamazepine, phenytoin or sodium valproate

---

Signs of complete trigeminal nerve lesion:

- Loss of corneal reflex
- Unilateral sensory loss of face, tongue and buccal mucosa
- Mouth opening leads to deviation of jaw to the side of the lesion

---

References

Grady KM, Severn AM. *Key Topics In Chronic Pain*, 1997. Bios Scientific Publishers, Oxford
Kumar P, Clark M. *Clinical Medicine*, 3rd edition, 1994. Baillière Tindall

The unconscious patient

An adult male is found collapsed at home with a decreased level of consciousness. He is brought to the accident department where his Glasgow Coma Score is 5/15.

What are the possible causes of his comatose state?

> An exhaustive list will not be required but a sensible and systematic approach looked for. You will need a system for categorising your answer. Listed below is one method. Another would be:
>
> ■ Trauma
> ■ Infection
> ■ Metabolic
> ■ Tumour
> ■ Drugs
> ■ Vascular – ischaemia/haemorrhage

> Consciousness depends on:
>
> ■ **Intact cerebral hemispheres**
> ■ A functioning **reticular activating system** in the **brainstem, the midbrain, the hypothalamus and the thalamus**
> **NB:** Focal damage to the cortex *does not* affect conscious level

Diffuse brain insult
■ Diabetic coma
■ Hyponatraemia
■ Hypoxia (due to respiratory insufficiency or blood loss, etc.)
■ Uraemia
■ Hepatic encephalopathy
■ Infection, e.g. meningitis
■ Post-ictal state

Brainstem pathology
■ Subarachnoid haemorrhage
■ Ischaemic event
■ Intracerebral bleed
■ Drugs (hypnotics/sedatives)
■ Tonsillar herniation
■ Compression by tumour

Midbrain pathology
■ Compression by supratentorial mass

Trauma leads to loss of consciousness by global ischaemic damage (e.g. extradural haematoma causing raised ICP and decreased CPP) or by pressure on the brainstem.

How would you manage this patient in the accident department?

- ABC approach to **resuscitation**

   With a GCS of 5, the patient is comatose (GCS≤8) and not able to protect his airway. He should therefore be intubated and ventilated. Treatment should aim to prevent any secondary brain injury
- **History** from any family/paramedics/nursing staff. Ask about:

   Speed of onset (sudden onset suggests vascular cause)

   Self poisoning

   Trauma

   PMH, e.g. epilepsy or diabetes
- **Examination**

General	Pulse
	Blood pressure
	Respiratory rate
Neurological signs	Lateralising signs
	Pupillary responses
Infection	Temperature
	Neck stiffness
	Rash

- **Investigations** will be directed by the history and examination

Trauma	CT scan
Self-poisoning	Toxicology screen
Metabolic cause	Urea and electrolytes
	Blood glucose
	Arterial blood gases
	Blood cultures
Infection	Lumbar puncture

The diagnosis may not be immediately obvious and further tests for unusual conditions may be needed (e.g. thyroid function tests, porphyrins, serum calcium).

   This will not alter resuscitation and supportive treatment.

Uncontrolled hypertension

A 48-year-old male patient presents for day-case inguinal hernia repair. On arrival on the ward his blood pressure is 220/130.

What would you do?

The patient's blood pressure **should be rechecked** ensuring that the cuff size is correct. Ascertain whether he is usually normotensive. A blood pressure this high is pathological and not likely to be due to anxiety. However, it could be rechecked following an anxiolytic if it is deemed appropriate. It may be that he is already on antihypertensives but has not taken them recently.

This blood pressure is extremely high and raises the possibility of **malignant hypertension**. Other features of this include papilloedema, encephalopathy and end-organ damage. This is a medical emergency and necessitates admission to hospital and urgent antihypertensive therapy.

On rechecking, the BP is 200/120. Will you anaesthetise this patient?

No. The surgery should be postponed until the blood pressure is under control and an explanation given to the patient. He needs to understand the implications of having uncontrolled hypertension both in terms of having an anaesthetic and also the long-term health risks.

A medical history with regard to his hypertension, particularly looking for an underlying medical cause (found in less than 10% of cases) should be taken. The condition should be investigated and this would need to be co-ordinated through his GP. The GP should receive a letter outlining the results of any preliminary investigations and the treatment commenced.

> **Routine investigation of hypertensive patients:**
>
> ■ **Urine strip test for blood and protein**
> ■ **Blood electrolytes and creatinine**
> ■ **Blood glucose**
> ■ **Serum total: HDL cholesterol ratio**
> ■ **12-lead ECG**
>
> **(British Hypertensive Society guidelines)**

What are the problems of anaesthetising a patient with uncontrolled hypertension?

■ Cardiac ischaemic events (especially if LVH present on ECG)
■ Arrhythmias
■ Cerebral autoregulation reset (shifted to the right)
■ Exaggerated cardiovascular responses
■ Poor left ventricular relaxation (diastolic dysfunction)
■ Renal failure
■ Bleeding

How soon do you think you would be happy to anaesthetise this patient?

Treatment needs to be established and continued for **several weeks**.

The numbers may 'normalise' quickly but several weeks of therapy are needed to reduce the abnormal vessel reactivity. The patient could then be anaesthetised when the diastolic pressure is **controlled** at or below 90–110 mmHg.

A diastolic blood pressure of >110 mmHg is associated with exaggerated cardiovascular responses and increased peri-operative complications as outlined above.

Which antihypertensive medication would you prescribe?

An oral beta-blocker would be reasonable in this man if there were no symptoms or signs to suggest malignant hypertension.

The British Hypertensive Society Guidelines recommend initiating therapy with a thiazide diuretic or beta-blocker unless there are contra-indications or a compelling reason to use another agent. Guidelines:

BP > 160–199/100–109   Should be treated (non-pharmacological initially only if no evidence of CVS disease or end-organ damage)

BP > 140–159/90–99   Treat if evidence of established CVS disease or end-organ damage

Target BP should be about 140–150/85–90

Antihypertensive therapy recommendations:

Agent	Compelling indication
■ α-blocker	Prostatism
■ ACE-inhibitor	Heart-failure, LV dysfunction
	Type-1 diabetic nephropathy
■ Angiotension II antag.	Cough induced by ACE-I
■ β-blocker	MI, angina
■ Ca2+ antagonist (dihydropyridine)	Isolated systolic HT in elderly pts
■ Ca2+ antagonist (rate-limiting)	Angina
■ Thiazide	Elderly patients

References

Aglan M. *Handbook of Clinical Anaesthesia*, 1996. Churchill Livingstone, Edinburgh

Deakin CD. *Clinical Notes for the FRCA*, 1998. Churchill Livingstone, Edinburgh

Goldstone JC, Pollard BJ. *Handbook of Clinical Anaesthesia*, 1996. Churchill Livingstone, Edinburgh

Morgan GE, Mikhail MS. *Clinical Anaesthesiology*, 2nd edition, 1996. Appleton and Lange, Stamford, CT

Ramsay LE *et al*. British Hypertension Society guidelines for hypertension management 1999: summary. *BMJ*, 4 September 1999, Volume 319, p630–635

Valvular heart disease

Preoperative evaluation of valvular heart disease

- Determine severity of lesion – history, examination and investigations
- Haemodynamic significance – e.g. echocardiogram, cardiac catheterisation
- LV function
- Degree of end-organ dysfunction – pulmonary, renal, hepatic
- Concomitant ischaemic heart disease

What are the principles of anaesthetising a patient with aortic stenosis?

- Maintain myocardial oxygen supply (maintain SVR with α-agonist)
- Maintain normal sinus rhythm
- Maintain heart rate at 60–90 bpm
- Maintain intra-vascular volume
- Give SBE prophylaxis
- Appropriate monitoring – arterial BP, ST changes (CMV$_5$), ?PAFC, ?TOE
- Avoid hypotensive drugs, neuro-axial blocks
- 'Slow and tight'

Critical aortic stenosis exists when the orifice is less than 0.5–0.7 cm^2 (normal is 2.5–3.5 cm^2). This correlates with a trans-valvular gradient of >50 mmHg with a normal cardiac output. Note that a low gradient may indicate LV failure.

In aortic stenosis the left ventricle is **hypertrophied** (concentric) and **poorly compliant** resulting in diastolic dysfunction.

LVH increases myocardial oxygen demand while the supply is decreased as a result of high ventricular wall pressures compressing intramyocardial coronary vessels. Aortic diastolic pressure and normal heart rate must be maintained to promote coronary blood flow.

The poorly compliant left ventricle causes elevated LVEDP which impairs ventricular filling. Patients are therefore very sensitive to changes in intravascular volume. Filling by atrial contraction is extremely important (contributes 40% of ventricular filling). Loss of atrial systole may cause heart failure or hypotension. Avoidance of arrhythmias is essential (consider immediate cardioversion).

Patients may behave as though they have a fixed stroke volume. Cardiac output is thus dependent on heart rate. Bradycardia is poorly tolerated.

Principles of anaesthesia for aortic incompetence ('fast and loose')

- Eccentric hypertrophy, dilated left ventricle
- ↑ Oxygen demand due to dilated ventricle and ↑ work
- GA generally well-tolerated as ↓ afterload → ↓ regurgitation
- Watch diastolic (coronary perfusion pressure) – tends to be low
- Keep HR 80–100
- Avoid bradycardia as ↓ HR → ↑ LVEDP which may → failure
- Avoid ↑ SVR as → ↑ regurgitation
- Dopamine/dobutamine preferable to vasoconstrictors

Principles of anaesthesia for mitral incompetence ('fast and loose')

- Eccentric hypertrophy, dilated left ventricle
- Proportion regurgitated depends on LV afterload
- Dilated left atrium
- GA generally well-tolerated as ↓ afterload → ↓ regurgitation
- Keep preload ↓ (keeps LV volume ↓)
- Keep HR 80–100
- Avoid bradycardia as → ↑ regurgitation
- Avoid ↑ SVR as → ↑ regurgitation

Mitral stenosis is covered in a separate short question.

References

Deakin CD. *Clinical Notes for the FRCA*. Churchill Livingstone, 1998,Edinburgh

Goldstone JC, Pollard BJ. *Handbook of Clinical Anaesthesia*. Churchill Livingstone, Edinburgh, 1996.

Morgan GE, Mikhail MS. *Clinical Anaesthesiology*, 2nd edition. Appleton and Lange, 1996.
   Stamford, CT

Wolff–Parkinson–White syndrome

A 22-year-old woman is admitted for a routine hysteroscopy. She has a history of being admitted to casualty 6 months ago with palpitations.

This is her ECG at the time of admission to casualty. What does it show?

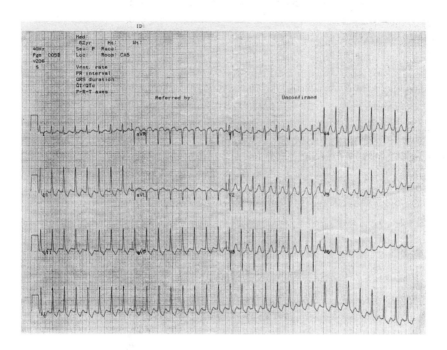

The ECG shows a supraventricular tachycardia. The rate is 190 beats per minute.

What would be suitable initial management if her blood pressure was stable?

■ ABC, oxygen, etc.
■ Check electrolytes (including Mg^{2+})
■ Carotid sinus massage
■ Adenosine – caution in asthma (causes bronchospasm) and if taking dipyridamole (prolongs half-life)

This is her resting ECG. What does it show?

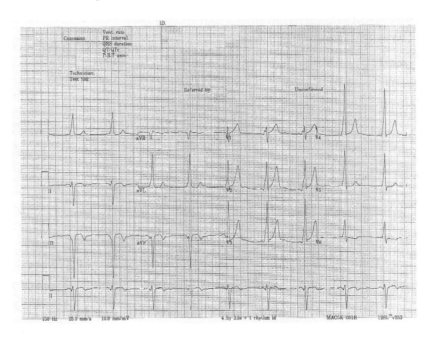

It shows sinus rhythm at a rate of 74 bpm. There is left axis deviation. The P–R interval is shortened (normal is 110–210 ms) and there are delta waves present. The diagnosis is Wolff–Parkinson–White syndrome. The ventricular complex is predominantly positive in lead V$_1$ suggesting Type-A WPW syndrome. (Type-B has predominantly negative ventricular complex in lead V$_1$.)

What is the 'delta wave'?

There is an **accessory atrio-ventricular pathway** (formerly called the bundle of Kent) which conducts the atrial impulse to the ventricles much faster than the A–V node. This results in the start of ventricular depolarisation sooner than normal, hence the short P–R interval. That initial ventricular depolarisation takes place in normal ventricular tissue (i.e. not specialised conducting tissue). The initial rate of depolarisation is therefore slower hence the slurred delta wave. When the rest of the impulse finally arrives through the A–V node, the specialised conducting tissue continues the ventricular depolarisation as normal so the rest of the QRS complex looks normal.

What are the implications for anaesthesia?

These patients may develop paroxysmal tachyarrhythmias during anaesthesia.
    Patients who have a history suggestive of frequent arrhythmias should ideally be investigated by a cardiologist and put on appropriate therapy. Those with infrequent episodes may not require any treatment.

What types of arrhythmia do they develop?

There are **two common arrhythmias in WPW**. These are **atrial fibrillation** (AF) and **A–V nodal re-entrant tachycardia**.

■ **Atrial fibrillation**
Patients with WPW who develop atrial fibrillation are at risk of very rapid ventricular responses as the accessory pathway does not provide any 'protective delay' like the A–V node. This may result in heart failure or may even deteriorate into ventricular fibrillation. In AF, most conducted impulses reach the ventricles via the accessory pathway so **delta waves are seen on the ECG**

■ **Re-entrant tachycardia**
A re-entry circuit is set up. After transmitting an atrial impulse, the A–V node usually recovers before the accessory pathway. If an atrial ectopic occurs at the right time it will transmit through the A–V node while the accessory pathway is still refractory. By the time it has done this, the accessory pathway may have recovered and the impulse will then pass through it back into the atria. As the impulses are all reaching the ventricles via the A–V node and not the accessory pathway, there are **no delta waves on the ECG**

How would you manage an intra-operative tachycardia?

■ **Treat possible triggers of rhythm disturbance** such as hypoxia, hypercarbia, acidosis, electrolyte disturbance or any cause of sympathetic stimulation
■ **Assess the degree of cardiovascular compromise**. If there was significant compromise then **synchronised DC cardioversion** starting at 25–50 J would be the treatment of choice. If the blood pressure was stable then the management would depend on the rhythm
■ **Pharmacological therapy**. For re-entrant tachycardia, adenosine would be the first choice. Class 1a drugs such as procainamide (5–10 mg/kg) and disopyramide prolong the refractory period, decrease conduction in the accessory pathway and may terminate both re-entrant tachycardia and AF. More conventional drugs such as amiodarone, sotalol and other beta-blockers such as esmolol may also be useful.

Are there any drugs you should not use?

Verapamil and **digoxin** are contra-indicated as they both preferentially block A–V conduction thereby increasing conduction through the accessory pathway. Although verapamil could, in theory, be used to terminate a re-entrant tachycardia its use is not advisable because these patients may then revert to AF or flutter. A further hazard with verapamil is that a tachyarrhythmia that *looks* like re-entrant tachycardia may actually be VT.

Adenosine would preferentially block the A–V node and therefore should not be used in AF.

References

Bennett D. *Cardiac Arrhythmias,* 1994. Butterworth-Heinemann, Oxford

Goldstone JC, Pollard BJ. *Handbook of Clinical Anaesthesia*, 1996. Churchill Livingstone, Edinburgh

Morgan GE, Mikhail MS. *Clinical Anaesthesiology*, 2nd edition, 1996. Appleton and Lange, Stamford, CT

Chapter 3

The Long Cases

Long case 1

'The one about the woman with a goitre for an emergency laparotomy'

A 75-year-old woman was admitted 24 hours ago with right-sided abdominal pain, nausea and vomiting over the last week. She has a past medical history consisting of a right total hip replacement 10 years ago and a CVA with right hemiparesis 4 years ago.

The surgeons wish to perform an urgent laparoscopy.

Drugs	Amiodarone 200 mg o.d.			
	Frusemide 20 mg b.d.			
	ISMO 60 mg b.d.			
O/E	Height 1.60 m, Weight 80 kg			
	Large diffuse goitre			
	HR 94 regular			
	BP 110/80 mmHg			
	HS I+II+0			
	Chest clear			
Investigations	Hb	9.7 g/dl	Na	132 mmol/L
	WCC	13.5×10^9/L	K	3.3 mmol/L
	Plt	189×10^9/L	Urea	12.2 mmol/L
	MCV	78 fl	Creat	110 µmol/L

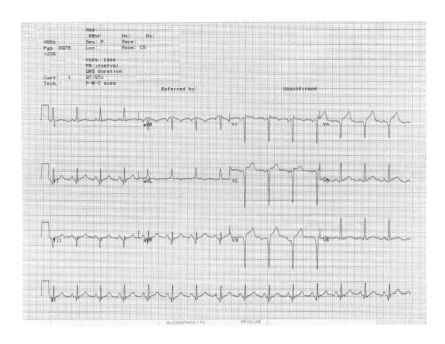

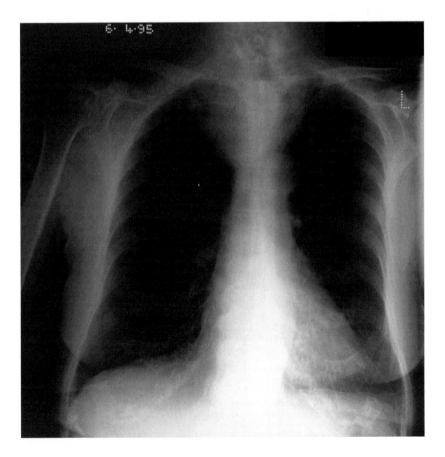

Questions

1. Summarise the case and the problems presenting to you as the anaesthetist.

This is an elderly lady presenting for emergency surgery with a significant cardiovascular history and a potentially difficult airway. She has been ill for the last week and may well be significantly dehydrated and septic. She will need careful resuscitation before surgery and a detailed assessment of her airway including imaging. The potential for a difficult airway and intubation is compounded by the high risk of aspiration. Surgery is urgent but not an emergency and these issues should be addressed before taking her to theatre.

2. Interpret the ECG.

The ECG shows sinus rhythm at a rate of 90 beats per minute. There are Q waves in leads II, III and aVF suggesting a previous inferior myocardial infarction. There are also Q waves in V_2, V_3 and V_4 indicating an old anterior infarction.

3. What does the CXR show?

This is a PA chest X-ray showing a large retrosternal mass with evidence of tracheal deviation to the left. The heart is not enlarged and the lungs are clear. Thoracic inlet views may help to image the lesion further but a CT scan would be ideal.

4. What is the mechanism of action of each of the drugs she is taking?

Amiodarone is an agent used to treat atrial and ventricular arrhythmias. It works by prolonging the repolarisation phase of the action potential (Vaughan-Williams class III). It also possesses some α and β-receptor blocking activity.

Frusemide acts at the thick ascending limb of the loop of Henle. It inhibits the cotransport of sodium, potassium and chloride into the medulla. The reduction in tonicity in the medulla results in the production of hypotonic or isotonic urine.

Isosorbide mononitrate is probably being used in this patient as anti-anginal therapy. It causes venous and arterial vasodilatation (venous > arterial especially at lower doses). Its mechanism of action is via the production of nitric oxide in the endothelial cells. This diffuses into the smooth muscle cells, activating guanylyl cyclase to convert GTP to cyclicGMP. The cGMP stimulates a reaction through protein kinases resulting in dephosphorylation of the myosin light chain and subsequent muscle relaxation (this may be by decreased free calcium concentration in the cytosol). The ultimate effects of nitrates are to reduce myocardial oxygen demand by reducing left ventricular end-diastolic pressure and wall tension. Coronary blood flow is also redistributed to the subendocardium.

5. Would you like any further investigations?

A CT scan of the neck and thoracic inlet is required to further assess the degree of encroachment on the airway. This will have significant implications for the conduct of anaesthesia.

Thyroid function tests (in particular TSH and free T4) would exclude thyrotoxicosis and the associated risk of thyroid storm under anaesthesia.

Given that the ECG suggests an old inferior MI and possible subendocardial ischaemia an echocardiogram may be useful to establish the resting ejection fraction. However, an echocardiogram gives no information about cardiac reserve. For example, a resting ejection fraction of 60% does not give any information about the ability to increase cardiac output. Of the numerous cardiac investigations available there are no consistently reliable indicators of cardiac risk for non-cardiac surgery except perhaps angiography.

6. How would you resuscitate her?

She has features that put her at high risk for postoperative mortality:

- Age > 65
- Presence of co-morbid disease
- Emergency presentation

She should therefore be transferred to an area where more invasive monitoring and resuscitation can be initiated such as HDU or ICU.

Her resuscitation should ideally be guided by the use of a pulmonary artery catheter. The aim would be to optimise her oxygen delivery with fluids and inotropes to obtain a supranormal value of 600 ml/min/m² according to current consensus of opinion regarding pre-optimisation of high-risk surgical patients.

7. Are you aware of any publications concerning pre-optimisation of surgical patients?

There have been a number of publications looking at the pre-operative optimisation of oxygen delivery for high-risk patients. They are based on studies showing that high-risk patients surviving major surgery achieved consistently higher postoperative oxygen delivery and cardiac index compared with non-survivors.

- **Shoemaker** showed the following values to be associated with survival:
  Cardiac index (CI)   4.5 L/min/m²
  Oxygen delivery (DO$_2$)   600 ml/min/m²
  Oxygen consumption (VO$_2$)   170 ml/min/m²
- **Shoemaker** et al in 1987 and **Boyd** et al in 1993 showed that producing supranormal values of oxygen delivery (>600 ml/min/m²) resulted in a reduction in postoperative mortality in high-risk surgical patients
- **Wilson** et al (BMJ, April 1999) studied pre-operative optimisation of oxygen delivery in major elective surgery. Three groups: conventional pre-operative care, fluid + adrenaline, fluid + dopexamine. Patients in the treatment

groups were taken to ICU/HDU at least 4 hours pre-operatively and arterial and pulmonary artery lines inserted. Fluids were given to increase the PAWP to 12 (average total fluid given = 1500 ml) after which adrenaline or dopexamine were commenced and increased until the target oxygen delivery was achieved (>600 ml/min/m²). They showed a reduction in hospital mortality from 17% to 3% (no difference between adrenaline and dopexamine groups) and a reduction in morbidity in the dopexamine group compared with adrenaline and control (fewer infective complications).

■ **A paper in *Critical Care Medicine*** in 2000 (prospective, randomised controlled trial of 412 patients undergoing major abdominal surgery in 13 hospitals from six European countries) compared the effects on morbidity/mortality of dopexamine infusion or placebo on fluid resuscitated patients. Patients were taken to ICU pre-operatively, invasive monitoring inserted and fluids given until set criteria met. Randomisation to dopexamine 0.5 μg/kg/min, 2 μg/kg/min or placebo followed. There was no statistically significant difference in 28-day mortality in the three groups although the authors speculated a trend towards lower mortality in the low-dose dopexamine group.

■ **Consensus meeting: management of the high risk surgical patient, April 2000**
  – Increasing global oxygen delivery in high-risk patients significantly reduces morbidity and mortality
  – In patients with significant ischaemic heart disease care needs to be taken to minimise oxygen demand
  – The earlier the intervention the better the outcome
  – Strategy should be as defined by Shoemaker's criteria for CI, DO_2 and VO_2
  – Low-dose dopexamine *may* have additional benefits

'Meta-analysis of the 14 published and three unpublished RCTs of perioperative optimisation of high-risk patients indicates that were the strategy generally adopted 11 lives could be saved for every 100 operations performed.' **Dr Owen Boyd**

---

8. How would you assess her airway?

Standard bedside tests for airway assessment such as the Mallampati score and thyromental distance need to be taken into consideration along with the CT scan appearances. An indirect laryngoscopy or fibreoptic nasendoscopy should be performed by an ENT surgeon to assess the likelihood of a good view of the larynx at direct laryngoscopy. However, an expected easy laryngoscopy does not imply a straightforward intubation in the presence of a large goitre. The site and severity of any obstruction should be established on CT scan (retrosternal goitre is midtracheal). The narrowest part of the trachea can be measured to guide the choice of tube size. It will also demonstrate exactly how far down the trachea the obstruction extends so that it will be known whether an endotracheal tube or tracheostomy will be able to get below it or not. In most cases it is possible to pass a size 7.0 tube beyond the obstruction and allow both the tube bevel and cuff to sit above the carina in a conventional way.

9. How would you manage her airway?

This woman is likely to have a full stomach even if starved and thus presents considerable aspiration risk.

If there is no evidence of tracheal compression on CT scan and clinically the intubation looks straightforward then a conventional rapid sequence induction and intubation could be performed. If the goitre is compressing the airway then a rapid sequence induction may be hazardous, potentially leading to loss of the airway in the event of a failed intubation. If there was no risk of aspiration then a gas-induction might be considered but this would not be appropriate here. An awake fibreoptic intubation, although not always the first choice technique, might be the technique of choice in this case.

10. What technique of awake fibreoptic intubation would you use?

> There are many ways to perform awake fibreoptic intubation. Having your own chosen technique and sticking to it will confirm to the examiners that you have performed the procedure many times before!

The procedure should be explained to the patient in an attempt to minimise anxiety(!). Intravenous access and standard monitoring is established. Premedication with an antisialogogue and a benzodiazepine/opioid would be given if necessary according to the clinical state of the patient. Supplementary oxygen should be administered via a face mask or nasal catheter. The patient may prefer the semi-upright position to being totally supine. Note that if there is a significant risk of loss of the airway then a surgeon experienced at rigid bronchoscopy should be present.

The nasal route is chosen in this patient for the sake of this question.

Five sprays of 10% aerosolised lignocaine is directed into the oropharynx at the start of the procedure (the nasal route should not stimulate the gag reflex).

The more patent nostril is chosen (ask the patient). The ET tube is lubricated and 'loaded' onto the bronchoscope. Topical anaesthesia and vasoconstriction of the nose can be achieved using 4% cocaine applied with cotton buds. The bronchoscope is advanced through the nose and pharynx with a 'spray as you go' technique using aliquots of 4% lignocaine injected through the working channel of the scope (alternatively, the ET tube may be passed through the nose before the scope). A jaw thrust manoeuvre will help to lift the tongue forward if it is obstructing the view. The cords and trachea are both visualised and sprayed sequentially. After a pause of 30–45 seconds the bronchoscope may be advanced into the trachea and the tube railroaded carefully over it. (Trans-tracheal injection can be used to anaesthetise the trachea but may not be feasible or advisable in the presence of a large goitre). The bronchoscope is withdrawn under direct vision to confirm the position of the ET tube above the carina. Once the tube is in place the induction agent can be given.

11. *What are the risks of laparoscopic surgery?*

> These have been discussed in the short case on laparoscopic cholecystectomy.

12. *How would you manage gas embolus?*

The surgeon should be informed and the abdomen deflated. Nitrous oxide, if used, should be discontinued. 100% oxygen is administered and fluid is given to increase central venous pressure. The patient may be turned into the left lateral and head-down position and the central venous line aspirated to try to remove gas.

References

Boyd O *et al.* A randomised clinical trial of the effect of the deliberate perioperative increase of oxygen delivery on mortality in high-risk patients. *JAMA* 1993, Volume 270(22), p2699–2707

Diprose P, Deakin MA. Fibreoptic bronchoscopy for emergency intubation. *International Journal of Intensive Care*, Spring 2001, p43–49

Farling PA. Thyroid disease. *BJA*, 2000, Volume 85(1), p15–28

Hagberg CA. *Handbook of Difficult Airway Management*, 2000. Churchill Livingstone, Philadelphia, USA

Mason RA. The obstructed airway in head and neck surgery. *Anaesthesia*, July 1999, Volume 54, p625–628

Report of consensus meeting: Management of the High Risk Surgical Patient, *International Journal of Critical Care Medicine*, 13–14 April 2000

Shoemaker WC *et al.* Prospective trial of supranormal values of survivors as therapeutic goals in high-risk surgical patients. *Chest* 1988, Volume 94(6), p1176–1186

Takala J *et al.* Effect of dopexamine on outcome after major abdominal surgery: A prospective, randomised, controlled multicentre study. *Critical Care Medicine*, 2000, Volume 28(10), p3417–3423

Wilson J *et al.* Reducing the risk of major elective surgery: randomised controlled trial of preoperative optimisation of oxygen delivery. *BMJ* April 1999, Volume 318, p1099–1103

Long Case 2

'The one about the man with pneumonia who needs a laparotomy'

A 42-year-old man presents with a short history of upper abdominal pain, vomiting and shortness of breath. The pain radiates to his right shoulder. The surgeons wish to perform a laparotomy.

PMH	Peptic ulcer disease His brother was admitted to intensive care with a high temperature following an appendicectomy
O/E	Sweaty, cyanosed Temp 38.2°C HR 120 SR BP 105/45 mmHg RR 25 bpm Reduced air entry at the right base with bronchial breathing

Investigations	Hb	15 g/dl	Na	149 mmol/L
	WCC	14×10^9/L	K	4.5 mmol/L
	Plt	380×10^9/L	Urea	11 mmol/L
	PCV	0.46 L/L	Creatinine	124 µmol/L

Blood gas on 40% oxygen:	pH	7.28
	PCO_2	31 mmHg
	PO_2	63 mmHg
	SBC	19 mmol/L
	BE	(–5 mmol/L)

LFTs normal

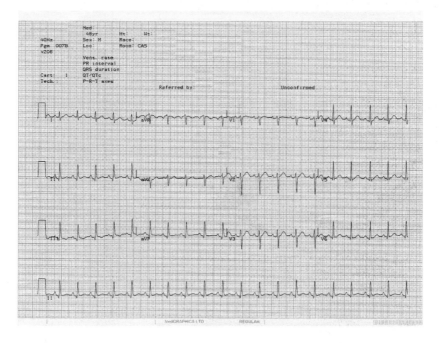

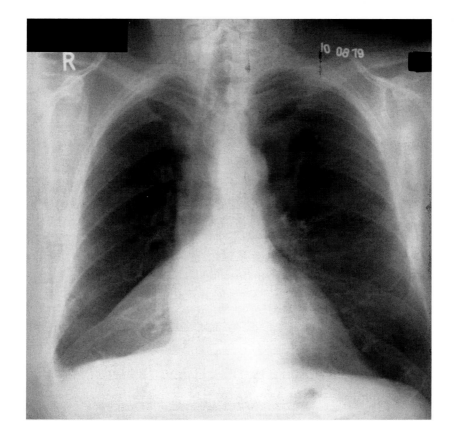

Questions

1. Can you summarise the case?

This man presents with a short history of abdominal pain and vomiting with a history of peptic ulcer disease but also has significant signs suggestive of an acute respiratory illness. There may be dual pathology. He appears septic, dehydrated and hypoxaemic. Of note in the anaesthetic history is what may have been a malignant hyperthermia reaction occurring in his brother and this should be thoroughly explored in the history and his brother's case notes if necessary.

2. What do you think about the chest X-ray and ECG?

This is a PA chest X-ray. There is shadowing in the right lower zone. There is also loss of definition of the right hemidiaphragm. The horizontal fissure is pulled down. These appearances are suggestive of right lower lobe collapse/consolidation. Given the clinical history this is most likely to represent pneumonia.

The ECG shows a sinus tachycardia of 120 beats per minute. There are no other abnormalities.

X-ray features of right lower lobe collapse:
- Well-demarcated shadowing/opacity in right lower zone
- Loss of right medial hemidiaphragm behind the heart
- Horizontal fissure displaced downwards
- Right heart border still seen

3. Tell me about the gases.

He is hypoxaemic on 40% oxygen. There is a metabolic acidosis with partial respiratory compensation.

4. What is meant by the term 'cyanosis'?

Cyanosis is a bluish discolouration of the skin (peripheral) or mucous membranes (central). It is seen when there are more than 5g/dl of deoxygenated haemoglobin in the blood. Central cyanosis is caused by cardiac or respiratory disorders and may improve with the administration of oxygen (providing there is not a large shunt). Peripheral cyanosis is caused by vasoconstriction, stasis and increased oxygen extraction by the peripheral tissues.

5. What do you think about his volume status? Discuss.

As mentioned earlier, he is dehydrated. The evidence for this is the history of vomiting and the presence of tachycardia, high Na$^+$ and disproportionately high urea compared with creatinine. His clinical picture is one of sepsis (see box below) and this will cause a relative hypovolaemia. He needs fluid resuscitation before theatre. This would be best achieved in a high dependency or intensive care setting and may be guided by a CVP line, pulmonary artery catheter and cardiac output measurements if available.

SIRS and sepsis: Systemic Inflammatory Response Syndrome (SIRS) is a clinical condition with two or more of the following:

- Temperature >38°C or <36°C
- HR >90 bpm
- RR >20 bpm or $PaCO_2$ <32 mmHg
- WCC >12 × 10⁹/L or <4 × 10⁹/L

Sepsis is a cause of SIRS that requires the presence of infection.

---

6. What is the differential diagnosis of his upper abdominal pain?

Given his history of peptic ulcer disease a perforated ulcer is an obvious suspect. Other causes might include pancreatitis, acute cholecystitis or a common bile duct stone, hepatitis, a subphrenic collection or even abdominal aortic aneurysm. The abdominal symptoms may be related to the lower lobe pneumonia.

7. What may be the cause of his shoulder pain?

This is likely to be due to referred pain from irritation of the right hemidiaphragm (C3, 4, 5). The origin of this irritation could be above or below the diaphragm.

8. Are there any other problems of note from the history?

A major issue if he requires surgery is the suspicion of a malignant hyperthermia reaction in his brother. The management would be greatly influenced by knowledge of what took place. Therefore, a thorough review of his brother's case notes and a discussion with his brother and the GP if necessary is warranted. The MH unit at Leeds holds a database of all the patients tested for MH susceptibility. His brother's name may be on this list.

The suspicion is high from the history so if the diagnosis cannot be excluded it would be wise to assume the family to be MH susceptible and anaesthetise this man as such.

9. Summarise your anaesthetic technique for laparotomy in this man.

During the period of resuscitation preparations should be made to provide a safe anaesthetic for a patient at risk of developing MH. This will include a vapour-free machine and circuit and the avoidance of known triggers such as suxamethonium and volatile agents. An epidural would have been ideal for analgesia and to help with postoperative respiratory function but it should probably be avoided in this case as he is septic. He is at risk of aspiration at induction but suxamethonium cannot be used. The airway could be secured either by a modified rapid sequence with rocuronium (only if expected easy intubation) or awake fibreoptic intubation. Thiopentone, etomidate, propofol and ketamine are all safe induction agents. Anaesthesia can be maintained with a propofol infusion and opioids such as fentanyl, morphine or remifentanil. Dantrolene should be immediately available.

10. Where would you send him postoperatively?

Postoperatively he should be nursed on intensive care. He has multi-organ failure (respiratory, cardiovascular, renal and gastrointestinal) and is likely to become more septic following the 'second hit' of surgery. He will also need to be monitored closely for the development of malignant hyperthermia.

Long Case 3

'The one about the woman with a melanoma on her back'

A 60-year-old woman presents for wide excision of a malignant melanoma in the middle of her back. The surgeons would like her to be prone. She is hypertensive, a heavy smoker and has a chronic cough. She had breast surgery for carcinoma 10 years ago.

Drugs	Enalapril 5 mg o.d.			
O/E	Temperature 36.8°C HR 72 regular BP 165/105 mmHg HS I+II+0 BS Widespread crackles and wheeze			
Investigations	Hb	11.6 g/dL	Na$^+$	143 mmol/L
	WCC	10 × 10^9/L	K$^+$	4.1 mmol/L
	Plt	260 × 10^9/L	Urea	8.9 mmol/L
			Creatinine	148 μmol/L

PFTs				Post-salbutamol
	FEV$_1$	1.5 L	(predicted 2.6)	1.7
	FVC	2.3 L	(predicted 3.5)	2.5
	FEV$_1$/FVC	65%	(predicted 74%)	68%

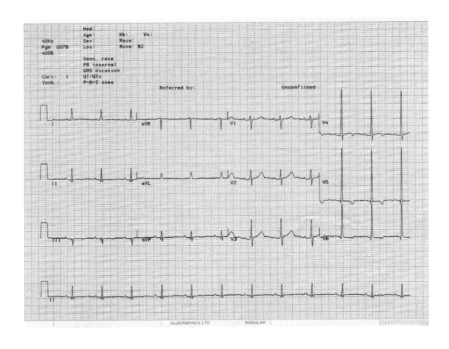

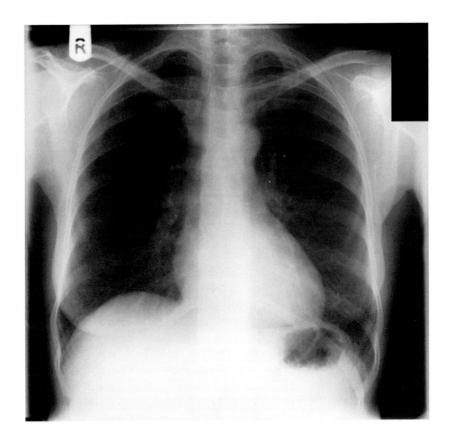

Questions

1. Can you summarise the case?

This lady presents for urgent cancer surgery that presumably cannot be performed under local anaesthetic for surgical reasons. She is hypertensive and has evidence of chronic obstructive pulmonary disease with a reversible component. She also has renal impairment. The preoperative assessment should concentrate particularly on optimising her chest and blood pressure before theatre.

2. Does the hypertension worry you? Why?

Yes. There is evidence of end-organ damage with the ECG showing left ventricular hypertrophy with strain pattern and the creatinine is raised at 148. Cardiac ischaemic events are more common in hypertensive patients with ECG changes of LVH.

3. What do you think about the chest X-ray?

This is a PA chest X-ray. There is asymmetry of the breast shadows in keeping with the previous left-sided breast surgery, the heart size appears normal and the lungs are clear. No metastases are seen.

4. What about the ECG?

The ECG shows sinus rhythm and a normal axis. There is left ventricular hypertrophy (sum of deflections in $V_2 + V_5$ >35 mm) and T wave flattening/inversion in the lateral leads suggesting left ventricular strain. This is likely to be due to long-standing hypertension.

5. What do you think about the creatinine?

As mentioned before this could be due to long-standing hypertension. It could also be due to enalapril if there is an element of renal artery stenosis. This should be investigated.

6. How would you interpret the pulmonary function tests?

There is a reduction in FEV_1 and FVC but also a reduction in the FEV_1/FVC ratio. This suggests an obstructive pattern of airway disease and the results after the administration of salbutamol show an element of reversibility. It is noteworthy that she is not currently on any respiratory medications such as a beta-agonist or steroid inhaler. She is also on enalapril which could be contributing to her chronic cough.

7. How would you anaesthetise her?

> Do not expect to be able to persuade the examiners that this can be done under local anaesthetic.
> That would make for a very short case!
> Perhaps just mention it in passing to make them aware you are thinking of the options.

Her chest disease and hypertension do not appear to be well controlled at present. Although her surgery is for cancer and therefore not truly elective, she would benefit from being postponed until better control of her chest and blood pressure have been achieved. A balance must be struck between the risk of postponing surgery and the risks of continuing when she is poorly controlled. Her chest could potentially be improved over a period of a few days by simple measures. She should be referred to a respiratory physician to optimise her chest with β-agonists, physiotherapy, steroids and antibiotics if necessary. The hypertension may require an increase in the dose of enalapril or the addition of another agent. Whilst it is recognised that under normal circumstances a period of several weeks is necessary to reduce the abnormal vascular reactivity associated with hypertension, she is only mildly hypertensive and it would not be appropriate to wait 4–6 weeks in a patient with a malignant melanoma.

On the day of surgery her ACE-inhibitor should be omitted. A benzodiazepine such as temazepam 20 mg and nebulised salbutamol 5 mg would be appropriate premedication. In addition to standard monitoring, intra-arterial blood pressure monitoring could be instituted before induction. Following preoxygenation and careful induction to minimise fluctuations in blood pressure an armoured ET tube is inserted and secured. Anaesthesia is maintained with nitrous oxide and isoflurane in oxygen. Her baseline respiratory function is relatively poor and the prone position will restrict lung expansion and increase airway pressures if not managed properly. Postoperative analgesia could be provided by combinations of paracetamol and morphine (via PCA if felt appropriate, e.g. large resection). Non-steroidals should not be used given that her renal function is not normal and she is already on an ACE-inhibitor.

8. What are the important aspects of prone positioning?

- Plenty of people to perform the manoeuvre – control of head, feet and two people on each side means a minimum of six required to turn the patient
- Patient is rolled with arms by the side onto the arms of two assistants
- Chest and pelvis are supported by rolls. Abdomen left free
- Respiration may be severely impeded if the abdomen is not free to move
- Head may be facing directly down or turned to the side
- Eyes should be padded and taped
- Care to avoid pressure on the eyes (blindness and supraorbital nerve compression reported) and downside ear

- Avoid pressure over preauricular area (facial nerve)
- Arms secured either by the side or in front
- Avoid brachial plexus damage by not turning the head too much, keeping the arms in a 'relaxed' position, not over-abducted at the shoulder. Protect the radial and ulnar nerves at the elbow
- Avoid excessive compression of genitalia and breasts
- CVS effects – usually well tolerated, may kink jugular vein. Obstructed IVC or femoral vein may lead to vertebral venous engorgement (problem in spinal surgery)
- ET tube must be well secured as must all lines

Reference
Stone D et al. The Neuroanaesthesia Handbook, 1996. Mosby Publishing, St Louis, Missouri, USA

Long Case 4

'The one about the man with hypertension and AF who needs a total hip replacement'

A 75-year-old man is scheduled for left total hip replacement. He was diagnosed with hypertension 2 years ago and recently developed dyspnoea on mild exertion. He takes dyazide, aspirin and digoxin.

O/E	
	Looks well for his age
	Weight 68 kg Height 5' 7"
	HR 80 irregular
	BP 180/105 mmHg
	Apex 5th intercostal space lateral to mid-clavicular line
	Ejection systolic murmur heard over precordium
	Breath sounds vesicular

Investigations				
	Hb	12.3 g/dl	Na	138 mmol/L
	WCC	8.9×10^9/L	K	3.6 mmol/L
	Plt	287×10^9/L	Urea	12.6 mmol/L
			Creat	170 μmol/L
			Glucose	7.8 mmol/L

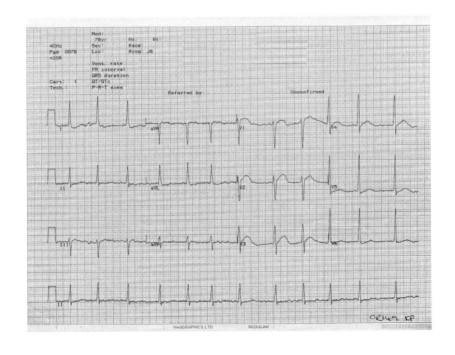

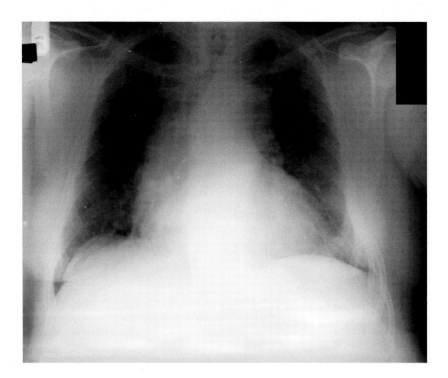

Questions

1. Summarise the case.

This elderly man presents for elective surgery with significant medical problems. He has hypertension, atrial fibrillation and evidence of left ventricular enlargement on the chest X-ray. He also has renal impairment. These problems need further investigation and optimisation before he can be safely anaesthetised.

2. Is he hypertensive? Is it controlled?

His blood pressure is 180/105. The British Hypertension Society (BHS) recommends that this level of hypertension is treated, as there are established cardiovascular effects. It is not adequately controlled as it is higher than would be recommended by the BHS and he has evidence of end-organ damage in the heart and kidneys.

> See the short question on uncontrolled hypertension.

3. Why does he get short of breath on exertion?

This may be due to left ventricular dysfunction secondary to long-standing hypertension. It may also be due to reduced cardiac output as a result of loss of diastolic filling secondary to the onset of atrial fibrillation (recent onset AF would account for the relatively new symptoms). Symptoms such as orthopnoea or paroxysmal nocturnal dyspnoea might give extra clues and should be sought. Left ventricular failure has a poor prognosis in terms of postoperative cardiac events. The presence of an ejection systolic murmur may be significant. It could be a flow murmur related to the hypertension but it would be wise to exclude significant aortic stenosis (although this would usually produce a lower pulse pressure). The shortness of breath could of course be related to another pathology such as COPD.

4. Look at the chest X-ray. Does he have pulmonary oedema?

The chest X-ray shows an enlarged heart with a cardiothoracic ratio of >0.5. There are prominent pulmonary vessels but no evidence of frank pulmonary oedema. There is unfolding of the thoracic aorta causing mild tracheal deviation.

5. Why is he on a diuretic?

This is most likely to have been commenced as first line treatment of hypertension by his GP.

6. How does dyazide work?

Dyazide is a thiazide diuretic that works by inhibiting the sodium-chloride cotransporter in the distal tubule. Excretion of sodium, chloride and consequently water is increased. Some of the sodium is reabsorbed from the distal tubule by exchange with potassium and hydrogen ions (hence the side effects of hypokalaemia and metabolic alkalosis). The exact mechanism by which thiazides exert their antihypertensive effect is not known. They do, however, cause a reduction in plasma volume, systemic vascular resistance and cardiac output.

7. Would that be your first choice of antihypertensive agent in this situation?

Thiazides are still the current first-line treatment of hypertension particularly in elderly patients but given that the control is poor the treatment should be re-evaluated. In the presence of cardiac failure an ACE-inhibitor would normally be justified but his renal function is abnormal. Renal artery stenosis would need to be excluded.

8. Why is he on aspirin?

This may have been commenced to reduce the risk of stroke as he is in atrial fibrillation and hypertensive.

9. Is that the most appropriate 'anticoagulant'?

No. For a man of this age in chronic atrial fibrillation the most effective treatment to reduce the incidence of stroke is warfarin.

10. Why is he on digoxin? How does it work?

He is in atrial fibrillation. Digoxin has direct and indirect actions. It acts *directly* by inhibiting $Na^+K^+ATPase$ in the sarcolemma cell membrane causing increased intracellular sodium and decreased potassium concentrations. The decrease in intracellular potassium causes a slowing of A/V conduction and pacemaker cell activity. The increased sodium concentration results in decreased extrusion of calcium and therefore a rise in intracellular calcium with a positive inotropic effect.

It acts *indirectly* by increasing central vagal activity.

> **Digoxin and hypokalaemia:** Digoxin competes with K^+ for a Na^+K^+ ATPase receptor on the outside of the muscle membrane therefore hypokalaemia potentiates digoxin toxicity.

11. Have a look at the ECG. What makes you say AF?

The rhythm is irregularly irregular and there are no discernible P waves. There is also evidence of left ventricular hypertrophy. The ST segments are depressed in leads I, aVL, V_5 and V_6 and the T waves are flattened. This may indicate left ventricular strain or may be a digoxin effect (not a typical 'reverse tick' appearance).

12. Is it controlled? How could you check?

The ventricular rate is around 70 beats per minute which appears to be controlled. However, resting heart rate is a poor predictor of rate control during exertion in atrial fibrillation. To assess the degree of control ambulatory ECG monitoring would be useful.

13. Would you anaesthetise him today? Why not?

No. He is listed for an *elective* major operation. His hypertension is not well controlled and he requires further investigation and management of possible left ventricular failure and his atrial fibrillation. Although the blood pressure 'numbers' may come down quickly the abnormal vascular reactivity associated with hypertension takes several weeks to settle down. The operation should therefore be delayed for this length of time.

A cardiology opinion and an echocardiogram may be beneficial to guide management.

14. What do you want an echocardiogram for?

An echocardiogram will help to assess his resting left ventricular function (not necessarily representative of cardiac reserve) and will exclude significant aortic stenosis or mitral valve disease. It may also reveal the presence of atrial thrombus secondary to atrial fibrillation. Formal anticoagulation followed by elective cardioversion to return him to sinus rhythm may significantly improve function.

15. His medical condition is optimised. He has no evidence of aortic stenosis. How would you anaesthetise him?

> As in many of the long cases there is probably no definite right or wrong answer here. You need to use a safe technique and provide sound reasons for choosing it.

If the atrial fibrillation is controlled (or ideally cardioverted to sinus rhythm) and his hypertension is controlled then the operation could be performed safely under regional or general anaesthesia. A spinal anaesthetic is appropriate if the surgeon is known to be quick enough. However, an epidural would be preferred, as it is less likely to result in marked swings in blood pressure, it will allow for prolonged surgery and it will provide ideal postoperative analgesia thereby reducing the stress response. There is now compelling evidence for the use of regional techniques where possible.

The evidence for regional versus GA

1. A paper in *Anesthesia and Analgesia* in November 2000 entitled 'Outcomes Research in Regional Anaesthesia and Analgesia' looked at a meta-analysis of 142 trials (9553 patients) comparing regional with GA for various types of surgery before 1997.
   Regional was associated with:
   - 30% reduction in overall mortality
   - 44% reduction in DVT
   - 55% reduction in PE
   - Reduction in graft thrombosis
   - Earlier return to normal GI function
   - 39% reduction in post-op pneumonia (48 RCTs)
   - MI reduced by 1/3 in 30 RCTs
2. A review in the *BMJ* in December 2000 looked at 141 trials including 9559 patients (before Jan 1997) where patients were randomised to receive intra-operative neuraxial block (epidural or spinal) or not. The authors concluded that:
   - Mortality was reduced by 30% in those allocated neuraxial blockade
   - The reduction in mortality was not affected by surgical group, type of blockade or where neuraxial blockade was combined with GA
   - There is a reduction in DVT, PE, transfusion requirements, pneumonia, respiratory depression, myocardial infarction and renal failure when neuraxial blockade is used
3. A clinical review in the *BMJ* April 2001 looked at interventions in *fractured hip*:
   - One systematic review of 15 RCTs (Cochrane review, 2000) showed reduced mortality at 1 month in the 'regional' group (borderline statistical significance). Not possible to conclude one year mortality
   - May be a reduction in DVT
   - Longer operating time with regional technique

- Summary… 'regional anaesthesia may reduce mortality in the short term after hip fracture surgery in comparison to general anaesthesia and may be associated with a lower rate of deep venous thrombosis.'

References

Gillespie WJ. Extracts from 'Clinical Evidence': Hip fracture. *BMJ*, 21 April 2001, Volume 322, p968–975

Rodgers A *et al.* Reduction of postoperative mortality and morbidity with epidural or spinal anaesthesia: results from overview of randomised trials. *BMJ*, 16 December 2000, Volume 321, p1493–1497

Wu CL, Fleisher LA. Outcomes research in regional anesthesia and analgesia. *Anesthesia and Analgesia*, November 2000, Volume 91, p1232–1242

Long Case 5

'The one about the young, thyrotoxic woman listed for a thyroidectomy'

A 31-year-old woman presents for a thyroidectomy. Three years ago she presented with tachycardia, heat intolerance and exophthalmos. She was diagnosed as having Graves' disease that proved to be unresponsive to radioactive iodine. She was therefore treated with carbimazole.

O/E	HR 120 regular
	BP 138/84 mmHg
	HS normal
	Chest clear

Investigations	Hb	13 g/dl
	WCC	15 × 10⁹/L
	Plt	170 × 10⁹/L

Urea and electrolytes normal

Albumin	37 g/L	
Calcium	2.23 mmol/L (corrected)	
TSH	0.17 mU/L (0.3–3.5 mU/L)	
Free T4	64 pmol/L (13–30 pmol/L)	

Thyroid scintogram – nodular thyroid

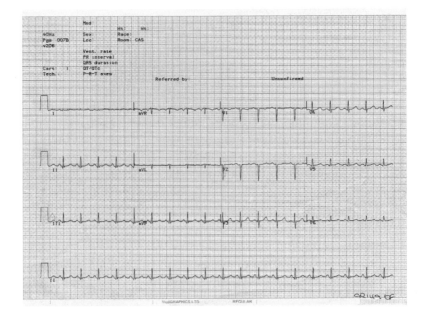

Questions

1. Tell me about the case.

This is a young woman presenting for elective thyroidectomy after failed medical treatment. There are two major issues that need addressing in the preoperative assessment.

She has been treated for Graves' disease but remains thyrotoxic. The operation must be postponed until she is euthyroid to minimise the risk of developing thyroid storm perioperatively. In addition, there is no comment in the history regarding the presence of a goitre and there has been no imaging of the thyroid to assess the airway such as a CT scan, chest X-ray or lateral thoracic inlet views.

2. Do you want any other investigations?

She should have the airway imaged as above. A plain chest X-ray will show lateral tracheal deviation or compression. Lateral thoracic inlet views will show compression in the AP plane. A CT scan will show both of the above and give additional information concerning the exact level at which the compression is occurring. It is especially useful with retrosternal extension of a goitre. Magnetic resonance imaging can give views in the sagittal and coronal planes if required. An indirect laryngoscopy should be performed routinely by the ENT surgeon preoperatively. It will give information on the quality of laryngeal view likely to be obtained at direct laryngoscopy and whether there is any evidence of recurrent laryngeal nerve palsy. Unilateral palsy results in ipsilateral cord adduction. This is associated with glottic incompetence, hoarseness, poor cough and aspiration.

Respiratory function tests (flow–volume loops) are of debatable value.

3. What are the symptoms and signs of Graves' disease?

> Signs of thyrotoxicosis have been described in the short case on thyroidectomy.

The signs of particular importance to the anaesthetist are atrial fibrillation, cardiac failure and cardiac ischaemia.

Signs unique to Graves' disease include the eye signs, pretibial myxoedema and thyroid acropachy.

The eye signs of Graves' disease are due to specific antibodies causing retro-orbital inflammation. The extra-ocular muscles are affected leading to a reduction in the range of movement. There may be exophthalmos, lid lag, lid retraction, conjunctival oedema and corneal scarring. These signs may be present even if the patient is euthyroid.

Pretibial myxoedema is a skin infiltration over the shins and thyroid acropachy consists of clubbing, swollen fingers and periosteal new bone formation.

4. How do thyroid hormones exert their effects?

The thyroid hormones T_3 and T_4 are transported in the blood mainly bound to plasma proteins. Their mechanism of action is thought to involve specific receptors bound to the plasma membrane, mitochondria and nucleus. The hormones enter the cell by a carrier mechanism after which most of the T_4 is converted to T_3. Binding of T_3 to specific receptors results in alterations in DNA transcription and thus protein synthesis and energy metabolism.

5. What do you think of the white cell count?

The white cell count is high. The differential count would help to distinguish the many causes. It would be important to exclude acute infection, the source of which should be found and treated before surgery.

Causes of a neutrophil leucocytosis:

- Bacterial infection
- Inflammation/tissue necrosis
- Metabolic disorders
- Neoplasms
- Haemorrhage/haemolysis
- Myeloproliferative disorders
- Drugs, e.g. steroids

---

6. How does carbimazole work? What are the side-effects?

Carbimazole inhibits the synthesis of thyroid hormones. It also has immunosuppressive properties. It may take up to 8 weeks to render the patient euthyroid after which it is continued at a reduced dose for about 18 months. Side-effects include rashes, pruritus, headache, nausea and arthralgia. The most serious side-effect is agranulocytosis (1/1000 after 3 months).

7. Would the surgeon be happy if the carbimazole had been continued up until the day of surgery?

No. Carbimazole increases the vascularity of the gland making surgical conditions more difficult.

8. Would you anaesthetise this lady today?

No. She should be rendered euthyroid before surgery and the rest of her investigations need addressing. She should also have the raised white cell count investigated and any infection treated.

9. What could be done to improve her preoperative state?

She could be changed to propylthiouracil for several weeks to see if she responds. In any case she should be commenced on a β-blocker to control the cardiovascular symptoms and signs.

10. Which β-blocker would you use and why?

Propranolol is the traditional β-blocker used to control the symptoms of thyrotoxicosis. It controls the cardiovascular complications and also reduces the peripheral conversion of T_4 to T_3. A heart rate of less than 85 has been recommended. Atenolol or nadolol are other suitable β-blockers.

11. She returns in one month well controlled. How would you anaesthetise her?

She should continue her β-blocker on the day of surgery and an anxiolytic such as a benzodiazepine would also be reasonable.

   The technique for securing the airway would be determined by the clinical findings and the results of the investigations of her airway. If a difficult intubation is expected then either gas induction or awake fibreoptic intubation is appropriate (intubation is difficult in 6% of cases of thyroidectomy). If there is serious concern that the airway may be lost after induction then awake fibreoptic intubation is the method of choice.

> The general principles of anaesthesia for thyroidectomy have been described in the short question on thyroidectomy.

12. She is on the femodene OCP. Would you stop it?

When a patient who is taking a combined oral contraceptive stops it there is a period of hypercoagulability before a return to baseline. It should ideally be stopped 4 weeks before surgery. As she has not already done so it should not now be stopped (BNF September 2000).

13. What else could you do to reduce the risk of thromboembolism?

The use of heparin and graduated compression stockings is recommended in the British National Formulary for women still taking the combined OCP and undergoing major elective surgery (and all surgery to the legs). In addition, pneumatic calf compressors should be used in theatre.

References
Farling PA. Thyroid disease. *BJA*, 2000, Volume 85(1), p15–28
Hagberg CA. *Handbook of Difficult Airway Management*, 2000. Churchill Livingstone, Philadelphia, USA
Morgan GE, Mikhail MS. *Clinical Anaesthesiology*, 2nd edition, 1996. Appleton and Lange, Stamford, CT

Long Case 6

'The one about the RTA with a flail chest'

A 35-year-old male has sustained multiple injuries in an RTA. He was the driver of a car hit by a lorry and the fire brigade spent some time extracting him from the vehicle. You are called to A+E to assist with the resuscitation and assess him for theatre.

Examination	Complaining of pain in right hip and chest
	GCS 15
	Intravenous fluids running, oxygen 15 L/min via facemask

	CVS	Pulse	115/min
		BP	85/40 mmHg

	Resp	Rate	40/min
		Paradoxical chest movement on the right
		Chest drains in-situ
	Positive DPL

Investigations	C-spine X-ray normal

Hb	11.0 g/dL
PCV	0.31
WCC	14.2×10^9/L

Sodium	138 mmol/L
Potassium	4.2 mmol/L
Urea	6.2 mmol/L
Creatinine	64 μmol/L
Glucose	11.4 mmol/L

Arterial gas on 15 L/min O_2	pH	7.20
	PO_2	9 kPa
	PCO_2	7 kPa
	BE	−11
	HCO_3^-	19 mmol/L

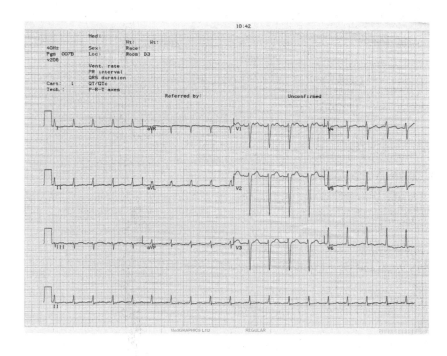

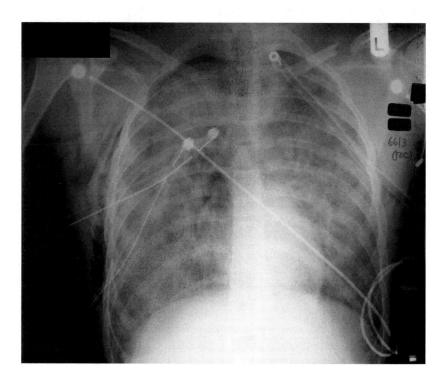

Questions

1. Can you summarise the case?

This is a 35-year-old man with severe multiple trauma who is still shocked and in need of further resuscitation. In particular, he has severe chest injuries with a flail segment, evidence of intra-abdominal haemorrhage, significant blood loss and a metabolic acidosis.

2. Tell me about the full blood count and arterial blood gases.

The full blood count shows anaemia with a low haematocrit suggesting there has been blood loss with (non-blood) fluid resuscitation. The white cell count is raised secondary to haemorrhage, acidosis and/or the stress response.

The arterial blood gases show a mixed respiratory and metabolic acidosis, in keeping with the clinical picture of a chest and lung injury along with untreated shock.

3. What are the causes of a metabolic acidosis?

The causes can be categorised according to the anion gap.

$$\text{Anion gap} = (Na^+ + K^+) - (HCO_3^- + Cl^-)$$

Normal anion gap is 10–18 mmol/L.

Metabolic acidosis – normal anion gap

- GI bicarbonate loss
- Renal tubular acidosis
- Ingestion of chloride-containing acids

Chloride tends to be retained as bicarbonate is lost

Metabolic acidosis – high anion gap

- Drugs*
- Lactic acidosis
- Ketoacidosis
- Uraemic acidosis

Bicarbonate is used to maintain normal pH

* The drugs responsible for a high anion gap include salicylates, paraldehyde, methanol and ethylene glycol.

Lactic acidosis is an important and common cause of acidosis. Normal blood lactate is 0.6–1.2 mmol/L and levels above 5 mmol/L cause significant acidosis. Concentrations greater than 9 mmol/L carry an 80% mortality rate. Lactic acidosis can be subdivided into type A and type B.

Type A lactic acidosis is the more common form, resulting from poor tissue perfusion and anaerobic glycolysis, e.g. shock, severe hypoxia, post-epileptic convulsion or exercise. The liver becomes unable to metabolise the high amount of lactate. Treatment is aimed at restoring the peripheral perfusion and oxygen supply–demand ratio.

Type B lactic acidosis is not directly caused by poor tissue perfusion. It is normally drug-related (biguanides, ethanol, paracetamol) but can be due to rare metabolic defects. These patients present with hyperventilation, vomiting, abdominal pain, drowsiness and coma.

4. *Where is lactate made?*

Lactate is made in skeletal muscle and red blood cells. When oxygen supplies are limited pyruvate is reduced by NADH to form lactate, the reaction being catalysed by lactate dehydrogenase. The importance of this reaction is twofold. It produces two ATP molecules and regenerates NAD^+ which sustains continued glycolysis in skeletal muscle and erythrocytes under anaerobic conditions. The limiting factor is the liver which must oxidise lactate back to pyruvate for subsequent gluconeogenesis. This pathway merely 'buys time' during periods of stress.

5. *Why is acidosis undesirable?*

Acidosis (respiratory or metabolic) is negatively inotropic and causes dilatation of systemic and cerebral arterioles. There will be a reduction in cardiac output and blood pressure.

Respiratory effects include hyperventilation (initially driven by the peripheral aortic and carotid chemoreceptors) and a right shift of the oxygen dissociation curve – Bohr effect. The latter will improve the unloading of oxygen to tissues but may impair uptake in the lungs.

Other effects include inhibition of glycolysis, hyperkalaemia, reduced consciousness and a leucocytosis.

6. *Tell me about the ECG and chest X-ray.*

The ECG shows a sinus tachycardia with a rate of about 110 beats per minute. There is minor ST depression in the lateral leads with T wave flattening. This may represent ischaemia related to cardiac trauma or secondary to severe hypotension.

The chest X-ray shows bilateral pneumothoraces with two chest drains on the right and one on the left. There are fractures of the 3rd, 4th, 5th and 6th ribs on the right and there is bilateral surgical emphysema with mediastinal emphysema visible at the upper right heart border. There is also a fractured clavicle and scapula on the left. The lungs are severely contused. Although it is not possible to demonstrate ribs fractured in two places on the X-ray there may be injury through the costochondral joints which would result clinically in a flail segment.

7. What is a flail segment?

This is due to severe chest trauma and occurs when a segment of the chest wall does not have bony continuity with the rest of the thoracic cage. The fractures at either end of the flail segment may be through rib or costal cartilage and therefore the diagnosis may be overlooked if chest X-rays are relied upon. The clinical signs are tachypnoea and asymmetrical chest wall movement with paradoxical excursion of the flail segment. Palpation may aid the diagnosis, feeling for abnormal movement and crepitus of rib or cartilage fractures.

Hypoxia results from a number of factors. Normal chest wall movement is disrupted, pain may limit tidal ventilation and there may be extensive underlying lung damage.

8. Why is he tachypnoeic?

He has a raised PCO_2 which is a potent respiratory stimulant.

Tachypnoea is also a response to shock as the body attempts to increase oxygen delivery to the tissues.

He has sustained a major chest injury with rib fractures, a flail chest and probable underlying lung injury. His lung mechanics will be altered, ventilation ineffective and gas exchange reduced leading to hypoxia. These will cause an increase in respiratory rate to try and compensate. In addition to this, pain will limit his chest wall movement forcing him to take rapid, shallow breaths.

9. How would you manage his fluid resuscitation?

This man is still shocked, most likely haemorrhagic in nature given the extent and detail of his injuries. He is tachycardic and hypotensive indicating that he has lost 30–40% of his blood volume (1.5–2 L).

ATLS classification of haemorrhagic shock

- Class I   up to 15% loss   Few clinical signs, replace primary fluid loss
- Class II   15–30% loss   Tachycardia, tachypnoea, decreased pulse pressure, BP low OR normal. Use crystalloid initially
- Class III   30–40% loss   As above plus low BP, anxious/confused. Crystalloid + blood
- Class IV   >40% loss   Life-threatening, rapid transfusion and surgical intervention

He needs swift assessment and management of Airway (with C-spine control), Breathing and Circulation, some of which has already been initiated.

Two large bore (at least 16-gauge) cannulae should initially be inserted with rapid infusion of 1–2 litres of crystalloid or colloid. Obvious bleeding from any external wounds should be controlled by direct pressure. Further management will depend on the response to fluid administration. This man requires:

- Blood crossmatched (type-specific if necessary)
- Central line
- Arterial line
- Urinary catheter
- Active warming and warmed fluids
- Cardiothoracic assessment
- General surgical assessment – he has a positive DPL
- Regular blood and blood gas analysis

Types of shock

- Haemorrhagic
- Cardiogenic   Myocardial damage, cardiac tamponade, tension pneumothorax
- Neurogenic   Often no tachycardia and normal pulse pressure
- Septic   Uncommon immediately after injury

---

10. Is he ready for theatre?

No.

He is still hypotensive and requires on-going resuscitation with repeated reassessment to address this. If, however, his condition were to deteriorate he may need a thoracotomy or early laparotomy as part of the resuscitation process.

References
ATLS Student Manual, 6th edition. 1997
Stryer L. *Biochemistry*, 3rd edition. Freeman, 1988
Weatherall DJ, Ledingham JGG, Warrell DA. *Oxford Textbook of Medicine*. 3rd edition. Oxford Medical Publications, 1996

Long Case 7

'The one about the chesty, obese man having a laparotomy'

A 60-year-old retired miner presents on your list for resection of a sigmoid carcinoma. He has long standing COAD with shortness of breath after walking 50 metres on the flat. He has had previous general anaesthetics with no problems.

Medication	Salbutamol nebuliser
	Salmeterol nebuliser
	Pulmicort inhaler
	Prednisolone – reducing regimen, currently on 2.5 mg qds

Examination	Obese
	Unable to lie flat

CVS   Pulse   120 bpm
        BP   150/90 mmHg
HS   muffled

Resp   Central trachea
      Hyperinflated chest
      Widespread wheeze
      Basal crepitations

Investigations	PFTs	FEV_1	0.88
		FEV_1/FVC	36% predicted
		PEFR	128 (predicted 439)

ABGs on air   pH   7.32
            PO_2 7.7 kPa
            PCO_2 6.8 kPa
            SBC   28 mmol/L
            BE   −1.2
            SaO_2 91% (air)

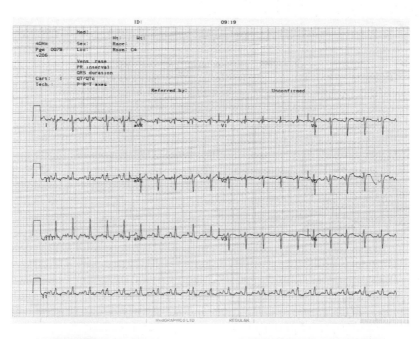

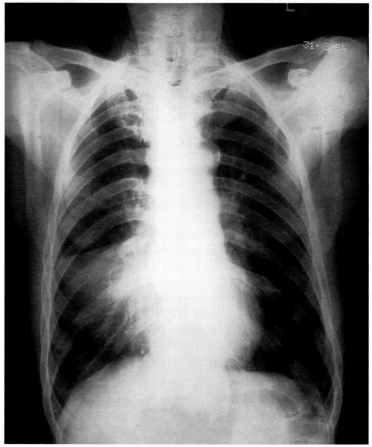

Questions

1. Can you summarise the main points in this case?

This is an elderly man with significant lung disease presenting for scheduled cancer surgery. His long-standing lung disease has resulted in concurrent cardiac changes and is compounded by a possible infective lobar consolidation. He is presenting for major abdominal cancer surgery and is at high risk of developing postoperative respiratory failure.

2. How would you differentiate between cardiac and respiratory causes of breathlessness?

A history of smoking or occupational risk factors with progressive breathlessness, cough and sputum production would suggest a respiratory cause while recurrent acute chest pain, palpitations, orthopnoea and paroxysmal nocturnal dyspnoea might suggest a cardiac cause.

Examination may reveal clubbing, wheeze and hyper-resonance (respiratory) or cardiomegaly, murmurs and a 3rd heart sound (cardiac). Raised jugular venous pressure and other signs of right heart failure may occur with both aetiologies.

> **Signs of right heart failure**
>
> ■ Raised JVP
> ■ Tender smooth hepatic enlargement
> ■ Dependent pitting oedema

Investigations may give further clues and should include ECG, chest X-ray, pulmonary function tests and echocardiography. If the diagnosis remains unclear, some form of cardiovascular stress testing may be indicated.

3. Can you comment on the ECG and chest X-ray?

The ECG shows a sinus tachycardia of 120 beats per minute and features consistent with right atrial and ventricular hypertrophy. (Right atrial hypertrophy results in tall, peaked P waves in II, III and aVF. Right ventricular hypertrophy results in right axis deviation, a dominant R wave with T wave inversion in V_1 and a persisting S wave in V_6.)

The chest X-ray shows large volume lungs consistent with long-standing chronic obstructive airways disease. In addition there is right middle lobe consolidation suggested by airspace shadowing in the region of the right middle lobe with loss of the right heart border and sharp demarcation of the horizontal fissure.

> **X-ray features of right middle lobe collapse**
>
> ■ Shadowing/opacity in right middle zone
> ■ Loss of the right heart border
> ■ Horizontal fissure displaced downwards
> ■ Diaphragm still seen behind heart

4. Tell me about the PFTs and ABGs.

The FEV_1 is severely reduced and the FEV_1/FVC ratio suggests an obstructive picture. There is no information about his effort during the pulmonary function tests. An FEV_1 of less than 1 litre is likely to result in postoperative respiratory difficulties such as sputum retention particularly as he will be having a laparotomy incision. His chest may be partially improved with treatment of the pneumonia.

The blood gas shows hypoxaemia with a mixed metabolic and respiratory acidosis. The bicarbonate is high–normal but may be higher than that when he is 'well'.

5. Are there any problems with steroids?

Yes. There are known side-effects from long term steroid administration including:

■ Osteoporosis
■ Hypertension
■ Peptic ulcer disease
■ Pancreatitis
■ Growth retardation
■ Central obesity
■ Cataracts
■ Easy bruising
■ Thin skin
■ Psychiatric effects (especially mania)

Particular side-effects of interest around the time of surgery and anaesthesia are immunosuppression, diminished wound healing, interaction with non-depolarising muscle relaxants (resistance to pancuronium), altered glucose tolerance, fluid retention and myopathy.

The other consideration with steroids is the perioperative regimen to use. A review article in *Anaesthesia* in November 1998 gave suggested treatment regimens:

Perioperative steroid regimes:

Patient currently on steroids

■ <10 mg/day	no additional cover
■ >10 mg/day + minor surgery	25 mg hydrocortisone on induction
■ >10 mg/day + moderate surgery	above plus 100 mg/day for 24 hours
■ >10 mg/day + major surgery	above plus 100 mg/day for 72 hours

Patient stopped taking steroids

■ <3 months	Treat as if on steroids
■ >3 months	No perioperative steroids required

6. Will you anaesthetise this patient on your list today?

No. His lung function should be improved as much as possible prior to surgery. He has right middle lobe consolidation, which needs treatment and further investigation to exclude a primary bronchial neoplasm or metastatic deposit. He also requires further basic investigations including a full blood count, urea and electrolytes.

7. How might you improve his condition prior to surgery?

He needs oxygen and regular physiotherapy with sputum sent for culture and antibiotic sensitivities. He should then be treated with appropriate antibiotics for a community-acquired pneumonia (determined by the hospital policy). He may require a flexible bronchoscopy by a respiratory physician.

A CT scan of his chest would help to exclude pulmonary metastases or a second primary.

8. All the above is done, no underlying lung tumour is found and his right middle lobe consolidation is treated. How would you anaesthetise him?

Oxygen and nebulisers should be prescribed preoperatively with careful consideration given to the potential side-effects of an anxiolytic premed. An intensive care bed should be booked for the postoperative period. Blood must be cross-matched and available in theatre.

With standard monitoring instituted in the anaesthetic room, an arterial line and epidural catheter should be sited prior to anaesthesia. The epidural may be commenced to ensure the block is both working and adequate for the proposed surgery.

The patient is preoxygenated and anaesthesia induced with propofol, alfentanil and vecuronium. An endotracheal tube is inserted and anaesthesia maintained with isoflurane, oxygen and air. A central line and urinary catheter are inserted.

In theatre, important considerations are oxygenation (ventilator settings, FiO_2, regular blood gas analysis), fluid status (CVP, urine output, pulse, blood pressure, blood loss), temperature control (warm fluids, HME, warm air blower) and maintenance of anaesthesia and analgesia.

9. At what level would you place an epidural?

This needs some discussion with the surgeon to establish what incision they intend to make. The epidural catheter should be sited near the dermatomal level of the midpoint of the incision, often lower thoracic. The choice may be limited by technical difficulties of siting a thoracic epidural.

10. What would your postoperative care focus on?

This patient is at high risk of developing postoperative respiratory failure and therefore needs close monitoring on high dependency or intensive care. The most important aspect of postoperative care is ensuring adequate gas exchange. Attention should be paid to:

- Humidified oxygen
- Analgesia without respiratory depression, optimally provided by an epidural. This should allow good tidal volumes and coughing to help prevent sputum retention and maintain gas exchange.
- Physiotherapy
- Bronchodilators
- Antibiotics

Other important elements include thromboprophylaxis, careful fluid balance and an assessment of nutritional status with total parenteral nutrition if required.

References
Kumar PJ, Clark ML. *Clinical Medicine*, 2nd edition. Baillière Tindall, 1990. London

Nicholson G, Burrin JM, Hall GM. Perioperative steroid supplementation. *Anaesthesia*, November 1998, Volume 53, p 1091–1104.

Long Case 8

'The one about the old lady with a fractured humerus'

An 81-year-old lady is admitted to A + E with a supracondylar fracture of her right humerus. The orthopaedic surgeons have put her on the emergency list for an open reduction and internal fixation.

Past medical history	Hypertension for 10 years. Mastectomy 8 years ago for carcinoma of the breast. Diagnosed as hypothyroid 6 months ago. For the past 3 weeks she has complained of severe back pain radiating to the right side of the chest and is due to be seen by a pain specialist.
Medication	Atenolol 50 mg/day Thyroxine 100 μg/day
On examination	She is conscious but breathless and pale. Temperature 36.6°C CVS: Pulse 85/min, regular BP 110/70 mmHg Apex not easily palpated HS quiet Mild ankle oedema Chest: reduced air entry on the left side

Investigations				
Hb	9.9 g/dL	Sodium	137 mmol/L
MCV	90 fl	Potassium	3.9 mmol/L
WCC	7.3×10^9/L	Urea	10.7 mmol/L
Platelets	208×10^9/L	Creatinine	57 μmol/L
		Glucose	8.0 mmol/L

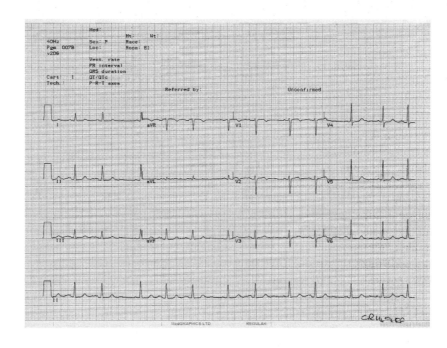

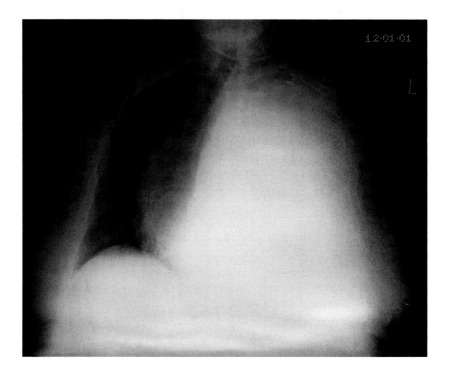

Questions

1. Can you summarise this case?

This is an elderly lady with a huge left-sided pleural effusion, possibly secondary to a recurrent breast carcinoma. She is also anaemic and hypertensive. She has presented with a supracondylar fracture which may require urgent reduction and fixation if there is associated neurovascular injury.

2. What are the main problems this lady presents?

The main concern with this lady is her respiratory disease and the aetiology of her pleural effusion. She is breathless with reduced air entry on the left side and the chest X-ray shows a massive left pleural effusion with mediastinal shift.

She has a normocytic anaemia which may be due to an underlying malignancy (pleural effusion, possible pathological fracture and previous mastectomy), hypothyroidism or may be from acute blood loss following the fracture.

The other concern with this lady is her cardiovascular status. She is a known hypertensive on anti-hypertensive therapy.

Supracondylar fractures are associated with neurovascular problems. The brachial artery together with the median and ulnar nerves are at risk of injury and this may warrant urgent exploration. The need for urgent surgery may not give sufficient time for further investigations of her concurrent medical problems.

3. What are the causes of anaemia and how can you differentiate between them?

Anaemia occurs when there is a reduction in haemoglobin in the blood below the reference level for the age and sex of the individual. The aetiology may be classified either by the appearance of the red cells or by the underlying disease process.

Classification of anaemia by disease process		
1. **Deficiency**	Iron Folic acid B_{12}	
2. **Haemolysis**	Intrinsic	Sickle cell, thalassaemia, G6PD, hereditary sphereocytosis
	Extrinsic	Immune e.g. SLE, lymphomas non-immune e.g. DIC, drugs, infection
3. **Marrow failure**	Aplasia Suppression e.g. malignancy, drugs, infection Dyserythropoiesis e.g. myelodysplastic syndrome	

Classification of anaemia by red cell appearance

1. **Hypochromic microcytic** (low MCH, MCHC, MCV)

   Classically iron-deficiency
   ? occult GI or gynaecological loss
   Thalassaemia

2. **Normochromic normocytic** (normal MCV)

   Anaemia of chronic disease
   Acute blood loss
   Hypothyroidism
   Bone marrow failure
   Haemolysis

3. **Macrocytic** (high MCV)

   Megaloblastic — B_{12}, folate deficiency (MCV >110 fL)

   Non-megaloblastic — pregnancy, alcohol, drugs (MCV 100–110 fL)

   (a megaloblast is a cell in which cytoplasmic and nuclear maturation are out of phase)

General symptoms of anaemia include tiredness, fatigue and dyspnoea but in this age group it can manifest as angina, heart failure and confusion.

The various forms of anaemia can be distinguished by history, examination (glossitis, angular stomatitis, koilonychia, lymph nodes, splenomegaly, hepatomegaly) and investigations.

Look at the degree of anaemia on the FBC together with the MCV, MCH and MCHC. The FBC will also show the white cell and platelet counts which, if normal, suggest the anaemia is not due to leukaemia or marrow failure. Haemolysis and haemorrhage will produce a reticulocytosis (check haptoglobins, bilirubin, urobilinogen). Examination of the peripheral blood film may give further information. Other investigations may include serum folate, B12, iron, ferritin, or haemoglobin electrophoresis but will be dictated by the clinical findings.

4. Would you request any further investigations?

The extent of investigation into this lady's medical problems will, in the acute setting, be dictated by the degree of urgency of surgery.

Although the ECG is normal (sinus arrhythmia), there is little evidence available to estimate her exercise tolerance or response to cardiovascular stress. Ideally these should be tackled before anaesthesia. Any symptoms of ischaemic heart disease such as chest pain, shortness of breath, reduced exercise tolerance and palpitations should be specifically asked for. After the effusion is drained, a repeat chest X-ray would be needed to assess her heart size. If her heart was enlarged then echocardiography would give some indication of the (resting) left ventricular ejection fraction.

Ideally her thyroid function tests should be checked and thyroxine dose adjusted if necessary (although the results are unlikely to be available prior to surgery).

Of major concern is the cause of the pleural effusion and a CT scan may help identify whether she does indeed have metastatic disease in her chest.

5. Would you want to drain the pleural effusion before surgery/anaesthesia?

Yes. This is a large pleural effusion causing mediastinal shift and clinical symptoms. Draining the effusion will improve her respiratory function in the short term and may give a further clue to the underlying diagnosis. A chest drain should be inserted and connected to an underwater seal. The drain should be intermittently clamped after each litre has drained to prevent re-expansion pulmonary oedema. Pleural effusions may be divided into transudates or exudates according to the protein and lactate dehydrogenase content of the fluid.

> **Causes of transudates**
> (protein <30 g/L and LDH <200 IU/L)
>
> - Heart failure
> - Hypoproteinaemia
> - Hypothyroidism
> - Constrictive pericarditis
> - Meig's syndrome

> **Causes of exudates**
> (protein >30 g/L and LDH >200 IU/L)
>
> - Pneumonia
> - Bronchial carcinoma
> - Pulmonary infarction
> - TB
> - Others, e.g. SLE

6. How would you anaesthetise this lady?

Brachial plexus block using the interscalene approach would be a reasonable technique in this lady.

The **advantages** of this technique are that it avoids the need for general anaesthesia and ventilation, provides excellent intra- and postoperative analgesia (a catheter can be used), avoids excessive movement of the painful arm (compared with the axillary approach) and should have minimal impact on her cardiovascular system.

The **disadvantages** of this technique are the potential complications, i.e. vertebral artery puncture, pneumothorax, phrenic nerve palsy, subarachnoid puncture, recurrent laryngeal nerve palsy and Horner's syndrome. Not all anaesthetists perform this block regularly and therefore they may choose a different technique.

7. How would you perform the block?

Informed consent should be obtained. Full monitoring should be established and an intravenous cannula sited.

The patient is positioned supine with the head turned slightly away from the side to be blocked. Gown and gloves are worn and the skin is cleaned. The interscalene groove is located at the midpoint of the posterior border of sternomastoid, at the level of the cricoid cartilage. The patient may be asked to sniff to make the scalene muscles more prominent.

The skin is anaesthetised at this point and the block needle inserted, aiming slightly dorsal. A peripheral nerve stimulator is used to locate the appropriate site. A 'pop' may be felt as the fascial sheath is entered (1–2.5 cm). The syringe is aspirated and the local anaesthetic solution injected slowly with regular aspiration.

References
Kumar PJ, Clark ML. *Clinical Medicine*, 2nd edition. Baillière Tindall, 1990. London
Pinnock CA, Fischer HBJ, Jones RP. *Peripheral Nerve Blockade*. Churchill Livingstone, 1996. Edinburgh

Long Case 9

'The one about the obese woman with fractured NOF'

A 76-year-old woman (height 148 cm, weight 87 kg) is awaiting a left hip hemiarthroplasty following a fractured neck of femur. She has osteoarthritis and a history of chronic obstructive airways disease having smoked most of her life. She also gives a history of recent onset of chest pain, relieved by GTN spray.

She is complaining of pain in her hip.

Medications	Ibuprofen 1600 mg/day			
	Moduretic			
	GTN spray			
O/E	Temp	38°C		
	Pulse	90 bpm, regular		
	BP	160/95 mmHg		
	Apex impalpable			
	Quiet heart sounds			
	RR	20 bpm		
	Bilateral basal crepitations			
Investigations	Hb	8.4 g/dL	Sodium	132 mmol/L
	Plt	190×10^9/L	Potassium	5.1 mmol/L
	WCC	5.8×10^9/L	Urea	12 mmol/L
	MCV	105 fl	Creatinine	137 µmol/L
			Calcium	2.1 mmol/L (corrected)

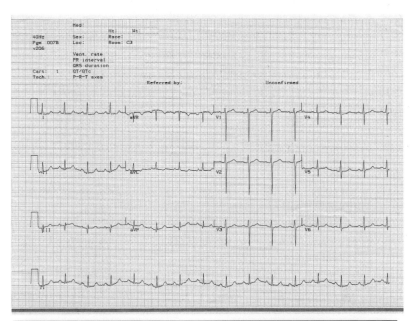

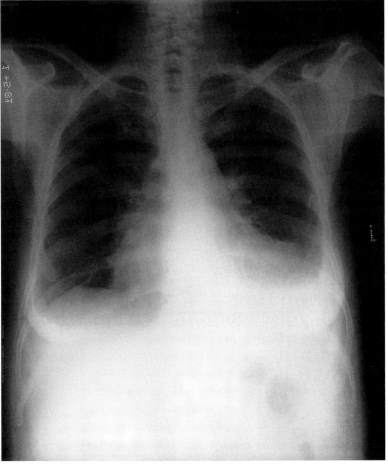

Questions

1. Can you summarise the case?

This is a 76-year-old morbidly obese lady with severe intercurrent medical problems who requires urgent surgery for a fractured neck of femur. The medical problems include:

- Ischaemic heart disease with current undiagnosed chest pain
- Possible cardiac failure
- Hypertension
- Renal impairment
- Chronic obstructive airways disease
- Macrocytic anaemia

These are the issues that need addressing during the preoperative assessment.

2. Would you like to comment on the chest X-ray and ECG?

The ECG shows sinus rhythm with Q waves in the inferior leads, suggestive of an old inferior myocardial infarction.

The chest X-ray is a PA film. The heart is enlarged and there are bilateral pleural effusions. The features are those of congestive cardiac failure.

3. What do you think about her weight?

Can you classify obesity?

She is morbidly obese with a Body Mass Index of nearly 40. A commonly used measure of obesity is the Body Mass Index. This is defined as the weight (in kilograms) divided by the height (in metres) squared. Morbid obesity is defined as a BMI > 35. The Broca index provides another measure of the degree of obesity.

> See short case on obesity.

4. Tell me about her anaemia.

What are the causes of a raised MCV?

She has a macrocytic anaemia, the more common causes of which would be vitamin B_{12} or folate deficiency, alcohol excess or liver disease.

> **Causes of raised MCV**
>
> ■ Megaloblastic   B$_{12}$ deficiency (commonly pernicious anaemia)
>   Folate deficiency (commonly nutritional)
> ■ Non-megaloblastic   Alcohol
>   Liver disease
>   Hypothyroidism
>   Reticulocytosis
>   Aplastic anaemia

5. *Would you transfuse this lady preoperatively?*

Her haemoglobin is 8.5 g/dL and although there is evidence that a haemoglobin of above 8 g/dL is acceptable, this is urgent surgery with a high likelihood of significant blood loss in a lady with known ischaemic heart disease. It would therefore be reasonable to transfuse her preoperatively being careful to avoid precipitating pulmonary oedema.

Hard evidence around the appropriate 'trigger' haemoglobin level for transfusion is lacking. The **ASA Task Force on Blood Component Therapy** issued some recommendations in 1996. They suggested that transfusion is rarely indicated when the haemoglobin is >10 g/dL but almost always indicated when <6 g/dL. Patients in the grey area (haemoglobin concentrations between 6 and 10 g/dL) should have their transfusion need assessed on an individual basis, weighing up the risks of transfusion against inadequate oxygenation. The recommendations are quite loose and the anaesthetist must use his/her clinical judgement.

A **paper published in *JAMA* in 1998** studied 8787 consecutive patients over the age of 60 years with hip fractures. Peri-operative transfusion in patients with haemoglobin levels of 8 g/dL or higher did not appear to influence the risk of 30- or 90-day mortality in this elderly population. At haemoglobin concentrations of less than 8 g/dL, 90.5% of patients received a transfusion, preventing meaningful interpretation of these data.

6. *What do you think might be the cause of her abnormal urea and electrolytes?*

There is renal impairment with a disproportionately raised urea compared to creatinine suggesting a pre-renal cause. Likely causes include dehydration or hypovolaemia secondary to haemorrhage. This could have been exacerbated by the use of non-steroidal anti-inflammatory drugs (inhibition of renal prostaglandin synthesis resulting in sodium retention and reduced renal blood flow).

The sodium may be low secondary to her diuretic therapy or could be due to cardiac or renal failure.

> **Common causes of hyponatraemia:**
>
> ■ Excess water   Renal impairment
>   Cardiac failure
>   Liver failure – hypoalbuminaemia
>   Inappropriate ADH
> ■ Sodium depletion   Intrinsic renal disease
>   Mineralocorticoid deficiency
>   Diuretics

7. Do you think her recent chest pain is significant?

Although the chest pain could be related to the ingestion of regular NSAIDs, the possibility of a cardiac origin cannot be excluded in view of her past history of myocardial infarction. The fact that the pain is relieved by GTN is not pathognomonic of a cardiac origin as oesophageal pain is also sometimes relieved by GTN.

A careful history must be elicited and may give further clues to the origin of the pain. Exercise stress testing to differentiate between the aetiologies is clearly not an option in this case.

8. Are there any other investigations you would like?

An echocardiogram will give some information about resting left ventricular function and the risk of postoperative cardiac events. A low ejection fraction (<35%) combined with a cardiac history and an abnormal resting ECG is predictive of post-operative cardiac mortality and would help determine the need for peri-operative intensive care. A normal resting echocardiogram, however, gives no information about cardiac reserve.

Although this lady has bilateral pleural effusions which could explain her tachypnoea, she also has a history of chronic obstructive airways disease. Pulmonary function tests will give an indication of the severity of her underlying lung disease as well as the degree of reversibility with bronchodilators.

In view of the raised MCV and hyponatraemia it would be worth checking her liver function tests and coagulation profile, particularly if a regional block is being considered. She may have liver disease.

Morbid obesity is associated with a higher than normal incidence of difficult airway which will need a full assessment and possibly further investigations.

9. How would you anaesthetise this lady?

This lady is a high-risk patient. She would benefit from preoptimisation with invasive monitoring, fluids (including blood) and possibly inotropes before theatre. However, there is also evidence to support the use of regional techniques at least in terms of short-term mortality and peri-operative events such as blood loss and DVT.

Choose your technique and back it up.

Two of the authors were examined on this long case. One gave a spinal anaesthetic and the other a general anaesthetic after preoperative optimisation with invasive monitoring. Both passed.

References

Carson JL *et al*. Perioperative blood transfusion and postoperative mortality. *JAMA* 1998, Volume 279, p199–205

Chen AY, Carson JL. Perioperative management of anaemia. *BJA*, December 1998, Volume 81, supplement 1, p20–24

Kumar PJ, Clark ML. *Clinical Medicine*, 2nd edition. Baillière Tindall, 1990, London

Louridas G *et al*. The value of the ejection fraction as a predictor of postoperative cardiac mortality in patients undergoing peripheral vascular surgery, 1992. *SA Journal of Surgery*, Volume 30, p12–14

Souhami RL, Moxham J. *Textbook of Medicine*. Churchill Livingstone, 1990

Long Case 10

'The one about the asthmatic child with torsion'

A 7-year-old boy presents with severe testicular pain (6 hour history) requiring urgent surgical intervention. He has been nil-by-mouth for 5 hours but has vomited in the last hour.

He has asthma with several previous hospital admissions for this. For the past 10 days he has had a cough.

Medication	Becloforte and salbutamol inhalers	
Examination	Weight 30 kg Pale, in pain and frightened	
	Pulse	145/min
	BP	105/60 mmHg
	Resp	widespread expiratory wheeze
Investigations	Hb	12.4 g/dL
	WCC	15.7×10^9/L
	PCV	0.38 L/L
	Sodium	137 mmol/L
	Potassium	4.1 mmol/L
	Urea	5.9 mmol/L
	Creatinine	54 µmol/L

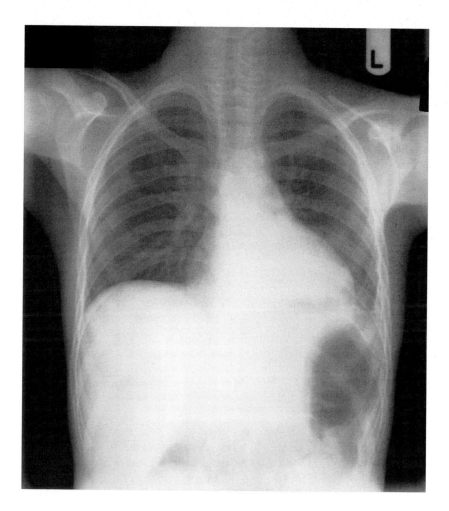

1. Can you summarise the case?

This case is a 7-year-old asthmatic boy presenting for urgent surgery. The important anaesthetic considerations are that this is an urgent paediatric case in which the child has symptomatic asthma, possible left lower lobe collapse/consolidation and requires a rapid sequence induction.

2. What is the differential diagnosis of testicular pain in this age group?

■ Testicular torsion	This results from rotation of the testis with interference of the blood supply and is usually associated with some abnormality. Venous compression from the torsion leads to congestion and eventual venous infarction unless corrected.

■ Acute epididymo-orchitis
■ Testicular trauma
■ Strangulated inguinal hernia
■ Idiopathic scrotal oedema

It is often impossible to differentiate between the first two diagnoses.

3. How urgent is surgery?

Surgery is urgent if testicular torsion is diagnosed or suspected. The torsion is corrected and the testicle fixed with anchoring sutures at the upper and lower poles. The other testicle is always explored and fixed in a similar fashion as this can occur bilaterally.

4. How would you assess the severity of asthma?

The history will elicit the duration of asthma symptoms, precipitating factors, frequency of attacks, increasing need for treatment and hospital admissions. The child's normal peak flow rate should be asked for.

On examination the respiratory rate, ability to speak, pulse rate and peak flow rate should be noted. The chest X-ray may reveal some pathology as in this case.

> See short case on asthma.

This child has significant asthma given the history of previous hospital admissions and a recent cough. He has widespread wheeze, a raised white cell count (which may be secondary to his surgical condition or from a chest infection) and left lower lobe collapse/consolidation on his chest X-ray. His respiratory rate, peak expiratory flow rate and response to bronchodilators need to be measured. He may benefit from preoperative physiotherapy if time permits.

5. Take me through the chest X-ray.

The chest X-ray shows blunting of the left costophrenic angle and loss of the left hemi-diaphragm behind the heart. Although there is not a classic 'sail sign' behind the heart, the features are consistent with collapse of the left lower lobe.

> **X-ray features of left lower lobe collapse**
>
> ■ Triangular opacity behind the heart (sail sign)
> ■ Loss of medial part of hemidiaphragm

6. What are the other important issues in the preoperative preparation of this child?

The important preoperative considerations in addition to assessment of respiratory function are:

- The preoperative visit which should focus on the parental anxieties as well as those of the patient
- This boy has been vomiting and therefore fluid and electrolyte status is important. An intravenous cannula should be in situ with appropriate fluid therapy commenced
- The patient's airway needs careful assessment as anaesthesia will involve a rapid sequence induction
- In addition to this, preoperative questions such as previous anaesthesia, allergies and loose dentition should be asked
- The patient and parents should be informed of the proposed method of induction and postoperative analgesic regimen
- Premedication may include bronchodilators and topical local anaesthetic cream if required

7. How do you assess and treat dehydration in children?

Distribution of water as a percentage of body weight				
	Premature	Neonate	Infant	Adult
ECF	50	35	30	20
ICF	30	40	40	40
Plasma	5	5	5	5
Total	85	80	75	65

Dehydration is commonly defined as mild (<5%), moderate (5–10%) or severe (>10%) and assessed clinically by decreased urine output, dry mouth, decreased skin turgor, sunken fontanelle (in babies), sunken eyes, tachypnoea, tachycardia, drowsiness and irritability.

Dehydration is treated by calculating the fluid deficit from reduced intake and insensible losses (vomiting, respiratory losses, sweating) and replacing the fluid and electrolytes needed. The hourly maintenance requirements should be calculated and added into the equation.

8. How would you anaesthetise this child?

In the anaesthetic room, ECG, blood pressure and pulse oximetry monitoring should be established. An intravenous cannula should be in situ. All drug doses must be calculated for a 30 kg boy and drawn up. The child's blood volume should be estimated (approximately 75 × 30 = 2250 ml for this boy) so that if blood loss is greater than 10% (225 ml), it can be replaced with blood. Appropriately sized endotracheal tubes must be available.

Following preoxygenation for 3 minutes, a rapid sequence induction is performed with thiopentone 150 mg and suxamethonium 60 mg. The trachea is intubated (6–6.5 mm ETT) and when the position is confirmed and the tube secured, cricoid pressure is removed. Anaesthesia is maintained with a volatile agent in oxygen and nitrous oxide or air. A non-depolarising neuromuscular blocking agent is added when the suxamethonium-induced block is wearing off.

A caudal epidural block can then be performed with the patient in the left lateral position and paracetamol suppositories inserted. For the caudal block 0.5–0.8 ml/kg of 0.25% bupivacaine would be suitable.

In theatre, anaesthesia is maintained as above. The boy should have core temperature measured with a nasal or rectal probe and should be actively warmed with a warm air blower. A suitable HME filter and warming blanket should also be used.

At the end of surgery, neuromuscular blockade is reversed and the patient extubated awake in the left lateral position.

Paediatric formulae:

Weight in kg	$(Age + 4) \times 2$
Tracheal tube internal diameter (mm)	$Age/4 + 4.5$ (if >2 yrs)
Oral tracheal tube length (cm)	$Age/2 + 12$ (if >2 yrs)

Maintenance fluid requirements (4 + 2 + 1 regimen)

0–10 kg	4 ml/kg/h
10–20 kg	40 ml + 2 ml/kg/h for each kg over 10 kg
Over 20 kg	60 ml + 1 ml/kg/h for each kg over 20 kg

---

9. What are the options for postoperative analgesia?

The options are opioids, local anaesthetic block, NSAIDs and paracetamol. Opioids may be given intraoperatively and continued postoperatively as an infusion or PCA if the child is old enough to manage it.

Morphine doses:

Child <6 months	i.v. loading dose	25–75 µg/kg
	i.v. infusion dose	0–20 µg/kg/h
Child >6 months	i.v. loading dose	100 µg/kg
	i.v. infusion dose	0–25 µg/kg/h

Diclofenac suppositories (1 mg/kg) are commonly used for postoperative analgesia but caution must be exercised in patients with asthma.

Paracetamol suppositories (initial dose of up to 40 mg/kg, then 15 mg/kg 6 hourly thereafter) are also used as co-analgesics with opioids.

Perhaps the best form of postoperative analgesia is from a local anaesthetic block, in this case a caudal epidural.

A caudal block is performed as an aseptic technique with gown, gloves and mask. The patient is positioned in a lateral position with the hips and knees flexed. The sacral hiatus is identified, flanked by the sacral cornua, and a needle is introduced through the skin and sacrococcygeal membrane. A 22-gauge needle or cannula-over-needle technique can be used. Once identified and after aspiration, the solution can be injected. It should inject with little resistance and there should be no subcutaneous swelling. The complication of dural puncture is more likely in children as the spinal cord ends at L3 but the dura ends at S3-4.

Long Case 11

'The one about the man for a total hip replacement with a history of previous DVT'

You are asked to anaesthetise a 62-year-old male for a right total hip replacement. He has been a smoker for 30 years and has ignored advice to stop. Consequently, he has a long history of respiratory and cardiac problems. He has had three admissions to hospital in the last year for chest pain and he becomes short of breath after walking 30 yards. He had a DVT 6 months ago, treated with warfarin for 3 months. He also has a small hiatus hernia diagnosed on CT scan.

Current medication	GTN tablets prn	
	Oxivent inhaler	
On examination	Weight	85 kg
	Height	5' 8"
	BP	140/80 mmHg
	HR	80 bpm
	HS	normal
	Auscultation of chest – widespread fine expiratory crepitations	
Investigations	Hb	15.0 g/dl
	WCC	7.0×10^9/L
	Plt	386×10^9/L
	Sodium	138 mmol/L
	Potassium	3.9 mmol/L
	Urea	5.2 mmol/L
	Creatinine	85 μmol/L

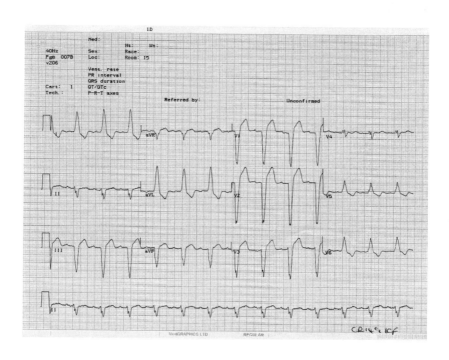

Spirometry		Ref	Pre Meas	Pre % Ref
FVC	Liters	4.00	3.21	80
FEV1	Liters	3.15	(1.01)	(32)
FEV1/FVC	%	76	(32)	
FEF25-75%	L/sec	3.40	(0.37)	(11)
FEF50%	L/sec	4.29	(0.30)	(7)
PEF	L/sec	8.12	(3.29)	(40)
MVV	L/min			
Diffusion				
DLCO	mmol/kPa.min	9.1	(2.2)	(24)
DL Adj	mmol/kPa.min	9.1	(2.2)	(24)
DLCO/VA	DLCO/L	1.75	(0.51)	(29)
DL/VA Adj	DLCO/L		0.51	
VA	Liters		4.27	

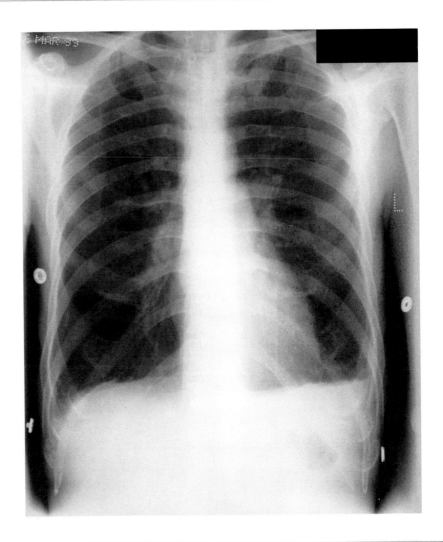

Questions

1. Present the history.

This 62-year-old smoker with severe COAD requires anaesthesia for a total hip replacement. He also has severe uncontrolled ischaemic heart disease and a history of DVT. This is an elective case, and because his symptoms are poorly controlled at present, he needs investigation and treatment of his cardiorespiratory problems before he is anaesthetised. He will also require attention to antithrombotic prophylaxis because the operation will put him at further risk of DVT and PE.

2. Discuss the significant findings.

The ECG shows left bundle branch block. This is likely to be due to severe ischaemic heart disease.

Causes of left bundle branch block

- Severe ischaemic heart disease
- Hypertension
- Aortic stenosis
- Acute myocardial infarction
- Cardiomyopathy

The chest X-ray shows hyperinflated lungs, flattened hemidiaphragms and generally coarse lung markings in keeping with long-standing COAD. The heart is not enlarged.

The PFTs show an obstructive picture with a markedly reduced FEV_1, a reduced FVC and a ratio of 32% suggesting severe airways disease. The reduced FEF_{25-75} is also in keeping with small airways obstruction. The transfer factor is only 24% of normal. He therefore has a diffusion problem and although the transfer factor corrected for lung volume is not much higher (as one would normally expect with emphysema) the clinical picture of many years of smoking combined with an obstructive picture on the other PFTs makes emphysema the likely diagnosis.

3. Is there anything else you would like to do before you anaesthetise him?

Further history regarding his episodes of chest pain would be very important in this case. If his pain was due to angina, he should be referred to a physician to improve his condition prior to elective surgery. He is not currently taking any antianginal medication apart from GTN tablets for symptomatic relief.

The presence of left bundle branch block on the ECG precludes further analysis. It is therefore impossible to say from the ECG whether or not he has suffered a previous myocardial infarct. An echocardiogram would show any wall motion abnormalities that might indicate previous myocardial infarction. It would also give an idea of his resting ejection fraction. If the ejection fraction is normal, however, this does not necessarily imply good cardiac reserve. An exercise ECG would not be possible in this patient so a dobutamine stress test or a thallium scan with dipyridamole would be more useful for assessing the potential for increasing cardiac output.

Arterial blood gas analysis on air would be helpful to further delineate his respiratory function and as a baseline with which to compare postoperative results.

It would also be important to establish the circumstances surrounding his previous DVT. If it was totally out of the blue, he may require a thrombophilia screen (protein C, protein S, lupus anticoagulant, antithrombin III and test for factor V Leiden mutation).

4. How do you distinguish cardiac from non-cardiac chest pain?

This is distinguished on the basis of the **history, examination and investigations**. Features of the pain that should be ascertained in the history are:

- Site and radiation
- Character (e.g. burning, stabbing etc.)
- Duration
- Severity
- Precipitating factors (e.g. exercise, emotion, movement or related to breathing or eating)
- Relieving factors (e.g. rest, antacids, GTN, etc.)
- Previous episodes
- Associated symptoms (e.g. sweating, palpitations, shortness of breath)

When attempting to diagnose the cause of a patient's chest pain, the history is likely to give the most clues. Further points that may be noted in the examination include:

- General features of vascular disease (e.g. hypertension, poor peripheral pulses, atrial fibrillation, etc.)
- Chest wall tenderness
- Pericardial or pleural rubs
- Pneumothorax

Investigations will be dictated by the preceding history and examination. Possibilities are (ranging from the simple to the more complex):

- ECG
- Chest X-ray
- Serial cardiac enzymes
- Troponin T
- Exercise ECG
- Gastroscopy
- V/Q scan
- Angiography

5. Tell me about regional blockade and anticoagulants.

The issue of central neuroaxial blocks and anticoagulation is one of risk versus benefit. Some of these risks and benefits are more quantifiable than others. Frequently the case is clear-cut, but there is a grey area in between. However, some guidelines are applicable.

In this country, the use of low molecular weight heparins (LMWH) for thromboprophylaxis is now very common. These drugs have some advantages over standard heparin:

- Laboratory monitoring of the anticoagulant effect is unnecessary
- No dosage adjustment is necessary
- They can be administered subcutaneously once a day

However, they also present some problems to the anaesthetist related to the timing of neuroaxial blocks. The half-life of LMWH is 2–4 times longer than standard heparin (and increases further with renal failure). This means that considerable anticoagulant effect may still exist in the 'troughs'. Relative overdosing of smaller patients could occur because the dose is not adjusted for the individual patient and the effect on Xa levels is not monitored.

The incidence of spinal haematomas has been greater in the US than in Europe. This may be a reflection of the fact that a twice-daily dosing regimen is used in the US (as opposed to once daily here) and therefore the troughs in plasma levels are not as deep.

Due to these factors, many studies have arrived at similar conclusions:

■ Single daily dosing results in a true trough in anticoagulant level that permits the insertion of neuroaxial blocks and catheter removal
■ Risk of spinal haematoma is increased with concomitant antiplatelet or oral anticoagulant treatment
■ Needle placement should be delayed until 12 hours after LMWH
■ The risk of spinal haematoma in patients with an indwelling catheter is increased if they receive LMWH
■ Catheter removal should take place 12 hours after LMWH or 1–2 hours before the next dose
■ The neurological state of the patient must be monitored

In this case, a regional technique would offer the advantages of improved outcome, reduced surgical blood loss, a decreased incidence of DVT and less interference with respiratory function. The patient is not anticoagulated at the present time and therefore a spinal or epidural is not contraindicated on this basis. The regional block must be appropriately timed between doses of prophylactic subcutaneous heparin in order to maintain adequate prophylactic cover whilst minimising the risk of spinal/epidural haematoma.

> In the final FRCA, questions about preoptimisation and the benefits of regional versus general anaesthesia have been asked in relation to this case. These topics are covered elsewhere in the long cases and are therefore not repeated here.

References

Horlocker TT, Wedel DJ. Spinal and epidural blockade and perioperative low molecular weight heparin: smooth sailing on the Titanic. *Anesth Analg*. 1998, Volume 86, p1153–1156

Kumar PJ, Clark ML. *Clinical Medicine*, 2nd edition. Baillière Tindall, 1990, London

Long Case 12

'The one about the diabetic man for TURP'

A 70-year-old man presents for a TURP. He has a past history of a shadow on his lung treated with drugs and irradiation. He is an ex-smoker (smoked for 20 years), gets breathless on exertion and takes glibenclamide for NIDDM.

On examination	Heart rate	90 bpm
	BP	180/90 mmHg
	Chest clear	
	Bladder distended	
Investigations	Sodium	141 mmol/L
	Potassium	4.2 mmol/L
	Urea	10 mmol/L
	Creatinine	190 µmol/L
	Blood sugar (random)	10 mmol/L
	Hb	158 g/L
	WCC	8.3×10^9/L
	Platelets	240×10^9/L
	Calcium	normal
	LFTs	normal
PFTs	FEV_1	1.5 L (predicted = 3.0 L)
	FVC	2.8 L (predicted = 3.9 L)
	FEV_1/FVC	54%
	DL_{CO}	76% predicted
	K_{CO}	79% predicted

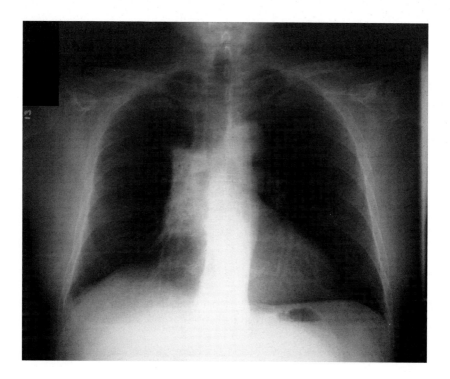

Questions

1. Summarise this patient's problems.

This elderly diabetic patient requires an anaesthetic for a TURP. He has significant respiratory pathology and renal impairment. As he is diabetic and has smoked heavily in the past he may well have ischaemic heart disease (which may be covert due to diabetes), cerebral vascular disease and peripheral vascular disease.

2. What could account for the biochemical results?

The urea and creatinine are both raised indicating renal impairment. His potassium and sodium are normal (important because of the risk of hyponatraemia due to TUR syndrome). The impaired renal function is most likely to be due to obstructive nephropathy secondary to prostatic hyperplasia. Other possible causes include diabetic nephropathy and end-organ damage from hypertension.

His random blood sugar of 10 mmol/L is not significantly elevated. The WHO currently recommends a diagnosis of diabetes mellitus if a random blood glucose is greater than 10 mmol/L. This gentleman is already diagnosed as diabetic and the concern now is the degree of control of his blood sugar.

3. *What do you think of the pulmonary function tests?*

The FEV_1 is decreased as is the FVC. However, the FEV_1 is decreased more and the FEV_1/FVC ratio is thus 54%. This suggests airflow obstruction. The transfer factor (DL_{CO}) is reduced but not enough to suggest a major problem with diffusion. It may be related in part to the previous radiotherapy and chemotherapy. The fact that the transfer factor corrected for lung volume (K_{CO}) is not very different would support fibrosis rather than emphysema. Chemotherapy with agents such as bleomycin or mitomycin can result in generalised pulmonary fibrosis.

4. *What other information might you want?*

Further information from the **history** such as:

- Exercise tolerance/SOBOE
- Any change in respiratory symptoms recently, e.g. cough, haemoptysis or wheeze
- Symptoms suggestive of ischaemic heart disease (e.g. chest pain) or other vascular pathology such as peripheral vascular disease or cerebral vascular disease
- History of hypertension. Is his blood pressure checked regularly?
- When was he diagnosed with diabetes?
- Usual blood sugar control including out-patient attendance, GP follow-up and method of testing blood sugar level (urine or blood)
- Haemoglobin A_{1C}
- History of postural hypotension (suggesting autonomic neuropathy)
- Previous anaesthetic history
- Whether the patient can recognise when his blood sugar is high or low

The patient needs a **12-lead ECG** to look for evidence of previous myocardial infarction, ischaemia or LVH.

From the point of view of his pulmonary function tests it would be helpful to know if he had any **reversibility of airflow obstruction with β-agonists**, and if he had cooperated well with the test. Depending on the degree of respiratory compromise, a set of **arterial blood gases** on air should be obtained.

His current chest X-ray should be compared to a **previous chest X-ray**.

A **coagulation screen** would be useful if a spinal anaesthetic was being considered because some prostatic tumours can produce clotting abnormalities.

Further investigations (e.g. echocardiography) would be guided by the history.

5. *Describe the chest X-ray. What may account for this?*

This is a PA film showing right-sided perihilar shadowing. It is sharply demarcated in keeping with fibrosis secondary to radiotherapy. The heart is probably slightly enlarged as the CTR is just greater than 0.5.

We think the chest X-ray in the exam probably showed right upper lobe fibrosis compatible with previous radiotherapy. Other causes of upper lobe fibrosis include:

- TB
- Sarcoidosis
- Silicosis
- Ankylosing spondylitis
- Chronic extrinsic allergic alveolitis
- Progressive massive fibrosis

6. How would you manage anaesthesia for TURP in this patient? What drugs might you give intraoperatively?

Also see short case on anaesthetic management of the diabetic patient.

A spinal anaesthetic technique would be appropriate for this patient. The advantages of a spinal over a general anaesthetic in this situation are:

- Recent papers suggest reduced mortality with regional techniques when compared to general anaesthesia alone
- Earlier detection of TUR syndrome or bladder perforation
- Superior analgesia
- Less detrimental effect on respiratory function postoperatively
- Decreased incidence of DVT
- Decreased surgical blood loss
- Earlier detection of hypoglycaemia
- Decreased stress response resulting in better control of blood sugar
- Decreased postoperative nausea and vomiting
- No hangover from a general anaesthetic
- Earlier resumption of oral intake (advantageous in a diabetic patient)

If he was keen to have premedication, care must be taken to avoid respiratory depression. Administration of oxygen would be prudent.

As the patient is diabetic he should be first on the list having omitted his glibenclamide. This drug has a long duration of action and therefore the patient should have his blood sugar monitored regularly for hypoglycaemia. There is debate amongst anaesthetists about the best regimen for managing blood glucose in these patients. I would start a sliding scale of i.v. insulin preoperatively.

Once in the anaesthetic room, monitoring should be established, a peripheral cannula (at least 16 gauge) sited and a crystalloid infusion started. Lactate and glucose containing fluids should be avoided. With full aseptic technique, I would use 3.0 ml of 0.5% heavy marcain for the spinal anaesthetic having first anaesthetised the skin with 1% lignocaine. Ephedrine and/or metaraminol should be drawn up ready to treat hypotension should it occur. A sensory level of T10 should be the aim.

Oxygen should be continued intraoperatively and gentamicin (or other prophylactic antibiotic) administered. If the surgical resection is prolonged or bloody then intraoperative haemoglobin estimation will help to guide the need for blood transfusion.

Glycine irrigation fluid containing alcohol is available. An alcohol breath test can then be used to calculate the volume of irrigation fluid absorbed by the patient. Intraoperatively he may require some sedation depending on his level of anxiety. Propofol or midazolam may be titrated.

7. During the TURP the patient becomes confused. What may be causing this?

Possible causes are:

- TUR syndrome
- Hypoxia
- Haemorrhage
- Hypotension
- Cerebrovascular event
- Myocardial infarction
- Hypothermia
- Bladder perforation
- Septicaemia

8. Tell me about TUR syndrome.

The TUR syndrome represents a group of symptoms and signs that occur as a result of the absorption of large amounts of irrigating fluid. This fluid is usually 1.5% glycine which is slightly hypotonic and has good optical and electrical properties for transurethral surgery. During resection of the prostate, large numbers of venous sinuses may be exposed to the irrigating fluid, which is under pressure. The syndrome, which can be fatal, can present intraoperatively or postoperatively. The symptoms are due to fluid overload, water intoxication and sometimes solute toxicity.

Symptoms include:

- Headache
- Confusion
- Restlessness
- Dyspnoea
- Temporary blindness

Signs include:

- Cyanosis/decreased O_2 saturation
- Arrhythmias
- Fitting

■ Hypotension or hypertension (often hypertension initially followed by hypotension)
■ Bradycardia
■ Pulmonary oedema

Symptoms of hyponatraemia are likely to develop if the serum sodium falls below 120 mmol/L. Haemolysis can occur due to very hypotonic plasma. Hyperglycinaemia can cause central nervous system toxicity and cardiovascular embarrassment. TUR syndrome is also more likely to occur if the irrigation fluid height is greater than 60 cm and/or the resection lasts longer than 45–60 minutes.

Treatment should be instituted as early as possible and therefore early recognition is vital. Hypoxia must be aggressively treated and may necessitate endotracheal intubation. This may also be required to prevent aspiration due to a decreased conscious level. Fluid restriction and loop diuretics are used to treat the fluid overload. If there are symptoms of hyponatraemia, then hypertonic saline may be required. However, it must be given slowly to avoid exacerbating fluid overload. Central pontine myelinosis can occur if correction of the serum sodium is too rapid. Diazepam or phenytoin may be required to treat convulsions.

References
McAnulty GR, Robertshaw HJ, Hall GM. Anaesthetic management of patients with diabetes mellitus. *BJA*, July 2000, Volume 85 (1), p80–90
Morgan GE, Mikhail MS. *Clinical Anesthesiology,* 2nd edition. Lange, 1996, Stamford, CT

Long Case 13

'The one with the stridulous woman for oesophagoscopy'

You are asked to anaesthetise a 65-year-old lady who has been admitted for an EUA, laryngoscopy, oesophagoscopy +/- biopsy. She has a 2 month history of dysphagia, stridor and a choking sensation when supine. She has recently lost 12 kg in weight, and now weighs 57 kg. She had a myocardial infarction 7 years ago but apart from being a smoker (20 cigarettes per day), her other medical history is unremarkable. She is on no medication.

On examination	Mild inspiratory stridor	
	HR	80 bpm
	BP	170/100 mmHg
	HS	normal

Investigations	Sodium	148 mmol/L
	Potassium	3.9 mmol/L
	Urea	8.3 mmol/L
	Creatinine	119 μmol/L
	Hb	17 g/dL
	WCC	9.3×10^9/L
	Plt	236×10^9/L

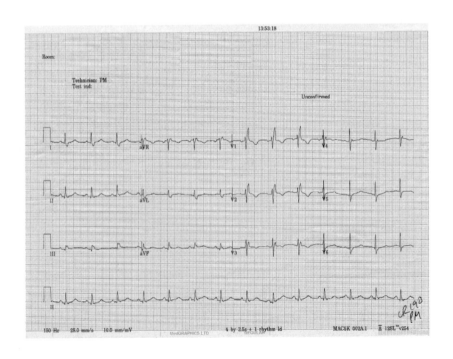

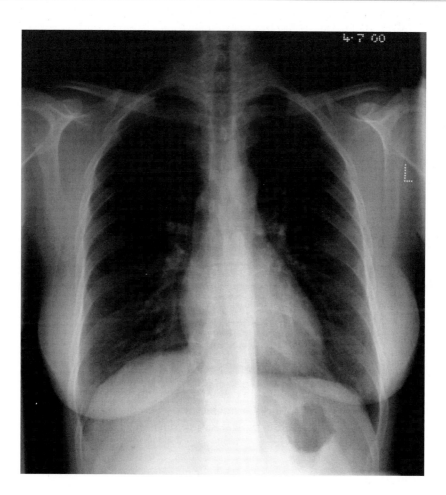

Questions

1. Can you summarise the case?

This 65-year-old lady, with a history of weight loss and stridor, has symptoms suggestive of a tumour that is partially obstructing her airway. The fact that she feels as if she is choking when she lies flat suggests the obstruction is severe. She requires an EUA of her oesophagus and larynx +/– biopsy of any lesion found. She has ischaemic heart disease, hypertension, polycythaemia and is also likely to have lower respiratory tract pathology because she is a smoker. Management of her airway will need careful consideration and consultation with the ENT surgeon.

2. What further investigations would you like?

Further investigation is important to help define the nature and level of the obstruction. The results of these investigations will dictate the anaesthetic approach to managing her airway. Helpful investigations would be:

- A **CT scan of her upper airway**. This will define the size and level of the obstruction. It will also help to suggest a diagnosis which will be relevant when considering if she is likely to need further surgery such as a laryngectomy
- **Nasal endoscopy.** If the glottis can be easily visualised in this manner then there is a good chance of being able to visualise the cords with direct laryngoscopy (providing there is no other anatomical reason why laryngoscopy would be difficult, of course)
- **Arterial blood gases**
- **Pulmonary function tests** including a flow-volume loop
- **X-rays of the thoracic inlet.** Not as useful as a CT scan

3. What are the possible causes of her symptoms?

Inspiratory stridor occurs when there is something partially obstructing the lumen of the airway. This may be arising from the lumen or the wall of the airway, or it could be due to extrinsic compression. This lady is a smoker and has suffered with considerable recent weight loss making the diagnosis of a tumour more likely. The tumour could be pharyngeal, laryngeal or oesophageal in nature.

4. Tell me about her ECG.

The ECG shows sinus rhythm with a rate of around 80 beats per minute and a normal axis. There is right bundle branch block given by the QRS complex being wider than 3 mm and the typical RSR pattern in lead V_1. The corrected QT interval is also prolonged.

5. What are the causes of RBBB?

- Normal finding in 5% of elderly adults
- Congenital heart disease   ASD
  Fallot's tetralogy
  Pulmonary stenosis
  VSD
- Respiratory disease   Cor pulmonale
  Pulmonary embolism
- Cardiac disease   Acute MI
  Cardiomyopathy
  Fibrosis of conducting system
- Other   Hyperkalaemia
  Antiarrhythmic drugs

6. How would you exclude a recent myocardial infarction?

A recent myocardial infarction may be identified by the history, examination and investigations available. This patient does not have hard ECG evidence of a past myocardial infarction (the exam ECG had inferior Q waves in addition to RBBB). If there were Q waves without ST elevation or T wave inversion it would only be possible to say that the infarct was older than a few days. ECG changes may have finished evolving after this time with Q waves developing and the ST segments returning to normal.

A recent history of sustained central crushing chest pain may help to date the infarct!

The cardiac enzyme changes may still be evident because the LDH can remain raised for 2 weeks. There are of course other explanations for a raised LDH.

Troponin T takes approximately 8 hours to begin rising and 12 hours to peak. It returns to normal within 5 days.

Recent onset of cardiac failure or an arrhythmia (e.g. atrial fibrillation) may have been precipitated by a myocardial infarct.

Other investigations such as echocardiography and thallium imaging can identify areas of abnormal movement or abnormal/absent perfusion but these tests are unable to date a myocardial infarction.

7. What are the causes of polycythaemia?

The causes of polycythaemia can be primary, secondary or relative. The secondary causes can again be divided into those with an appropriate increase in erythropoietin and those with an inappropriate increase.

Primary
- Polycythaemia rubra vera

Secondary (with an appropriate increase in erythropoietin)
- High altitude
- Respiratory disease
- Cyanotic heart disease
- Heavy smoking

Secondary (with an inappropriate increase in erythropoietin)
- Renal cell carcinoma
- Hepatocellular carcinoma
- Cerebellar haemangioblastoma
- Massive uterine fibroma

Relative
- Stress polycythaemia
- Dehydration
- Burns

8. What are the anaesthetic problems associated with hypertension?

See short answer question on uncontrolled hypertension.

9. *How would you anaesthetise this woman?*

The way in which this patient should be anaesthetised depends very much on the results of the investigations listed above. The nature and level of the obstruction are critical to the planning of the anaesthetic. If we assume that she has an obstructive lesion in or around the larynx then the first decision to be made is whether intubation is likely to be possible or whether the patient will require an awake tracheostomy under local anaesthesia. Whether or not the patient will ultimately require a tracheostomy for relief of symptoms will be an important consideration anyway.

These decisions should be made in collaboration with an experienced ENT surgeon who has performed a nasal endoscopic examination of the patient. This examination will show whether direct laryngoscopy is likely to be possible. If, with nasal endoscopy, the larynx is not visible and the anatomy is very abnormal then an awake tracheostomy under local anaesthesia should be performed.

If intubation is considered likely to be possible then an inhalational induction should be planned. This should take place in theatre with the ENT surgeon scrubbed to perform a tracheostomy if necessary. Other difficult airway equipment should be available to hand, including a rigid bronchoscope.

Sevoflurane or halothane could be used and laryngoscopy attempted when the patient is deep enough. It may still be prudent at this point to perform a tracheostomy if the patient is breathing spontaneously but the larynx is not visible on direct laryngoscopy. Once intubation is confirmed, a neuromuscular blocker could be given.

For monitoring this patient, an arterial line would be useful because of her hypertension (which is not controlled and the surgery cannot be postponed for 6 weeks until it is) and ischaemic heart disease.

Fibreoptic intubation in the patient with an obstructed airway

This can be hazardous for several reasons:

- ■ Altered anatomy causes loss of usual landmarks
- ■ Airway trauma can cause oedema and bleeding leading to total airway obstruction
- ■ Sedation and relaxation of the patient are difficult to achieve (and dangerous)
- ■ Emergency tracheostomy in an awake but hypoxic patient is very difficult

---

10. *What would your maintenance technique be and how would you manage her postoperative care?*

A remifentanil infusion may be useful for a stimulating procedure of short duration that is unlikely to require a large amount of postoperative analgesia. The rapid recovery from remifentanil is also desirable. In addition to this, sevoflurane in a mixture of oxygen and nitrous oxide could be used. This technique would hopefully give stable cardiovascular conditions. It is important to liaise with the surgeon during the procedure in order to know what the surgical findings were and what has been done to the airway.

Her postoperative care would depend on the operative findings and the difficulties encountered with her airway on induction and emergence. These factors would dictate what level of nursing care (i.e. general ward, HDU or ICU) the patient required.

As with any patient in the postoperative period it is important to pay attention to the points listed in the box below.

Questions on postoperative care:

When answering questions on postoperative care you should think about the following:

- Nursing dependency (ward, HDU or ICU)
- Pain-relief *and* anti-emetics
- Oxygen therapy
- Fluid therapy
- Physiotherapy
- Specific complications (e.g. post-thyroidectomy bleeding)
- Specific observations (e.g. neurological observations)

References

Kumar PJ, Clark ML. *Clinical Medicine*, 2nd edition, 1990. Baillière Tindall, London

Mason RA, Fielder CP. The obstructed airway in head and neck surgery. *Anaesthesia*, July 1999, Volume 54, p625–628

Long Case 14

'The one about the collapsed drug addict'

You are called to the accident and emergency department to see a 26-year-old male. He has been found semiconscious complaining of weak legs. There is a past history of intravenous drug abuse, depression and alcohol abuse. There is a vague history of heroin overdose.

On examination	He is agitated	
	GCS	13/15 after naloxone
	BP	80/40 mmHg
	Heart rate	56 bpm
Investigations	Sodium	135 mmol/L
	Potassium	7.9 mmol/L
	Urea	30.1 mmol/L
	Creatinine	352 μmol/L
	CK	43 000 U/L
	Hb	14 g/dl
	WCC	15×10^9/L
	Plts	255×10^9/L
	Blood gases on air	
	pH	7.2
	PO_2	8.0 kPa
	PCO_2	6.0 kPa
	HCO_3^-	19 mmol/L
	BE	−6

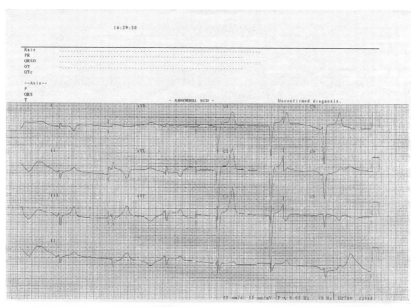

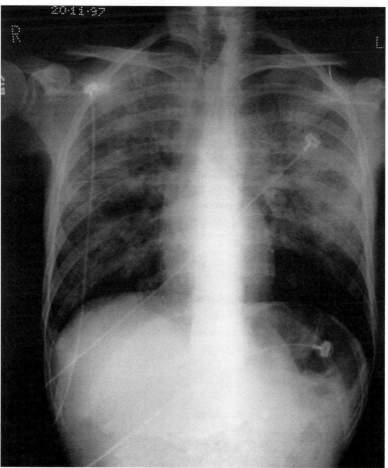

Questions

1. What are the possible causes of weak legs in such a patient?

The most likely cause of this patient's weak legs is muscle damage from rhabdomyolysis. Other possible causes are:

- The extremely high serum potassium level
- Polyneuropathy caused by drugs or alcohol
- Vascular injury secondary to injection
- Spinal cord damage from either compression (by tumour, blood clot or disc prolapse), infarction or trauma
- Guillain–Barré syndrome
- Vitamin deficiencies

Important points in the history will be whether the onset was gradual or sudden, and whether the limbs are spastic or not.

2. What do you think of the blood results?

The urea and electrolytes show that the patient is in acute renal failure. Both the urea and the creatinine are more than trebled. The serum potassium is very high and needs immediate correction as the patient is in imminent danger of suffering a cardiac arrest.

The creatine kinase is so high that this can only be caused by significant skeletal muscle damage (rhabdomyolysis). This destruction of muscle will have largely contributed to the raised potassium.

The full blood count is normal except for a raised white cell count. This suggests infection or an acute phase response.

The blood gases show a metabolic acidosis with poor respiratory compensation. The failure of the respiratory system to compensate may be due to a decreased conscious level and possible opioid intoxication. The metabolic component will be the result of rhabdomyolysis, sepsis (decreased perfusion) and renal failure. The patient is also hypoxaemic and this may be due to ARDS/sepsis.

3. What do you think the diagnosis is?

The diagnosis is rhabdomyolysis. High levels of myoglobin released from dead muscle have caused acute renal failure. Lying immobile on the floor for a long period of time may have caused the rhabdomyolysis. Hypotension and dehydration will exacerbate the damage. Other causes of rhabdomyolysis include cocaine abuse, alcohol (both chronic abuse and binge drinking), sepsis, prolonged fitting, electric shock or crush injury.

4. What effect does a raised K^+ have on the myocardium?

A raised extracellular potassium level causes a less negative resting membrane potential in the cardiac myocytes. The higher the potassium level the more fast Na^+ channels are inactivated. The action potential then becomes dependent on the slow (Ca^{2+}) channels, so the steepness and duration of the action potential upstroke become diminished.

The ECG changes include:

- Peaked T waves
- Widening of the QRS complex
- Bradycardia
- Atrial standstill
- Ventricular tachycardia and ventricular fibrillation can occur
- Sine-wave appearance
- Asystole

5. *What are the possible causes of the pulmonary oedema?*

The pulmonary oedema could be cardiogenic (although the heart does not appear enlarged on the AP film) or non-cardiogenic. ARDS is the most likely cause of pulmonary oedema in this situation.

Cardiac causes could be secondary to an alcoholic cardiomyopathy or sepsis causing poor left ventricular function.

6. *What would be your immediate management?*

It should be recognised from the outset that this patient is critically ill. He should be nursed in a high-dependency or intensive care area, such as the accident and emergency resuscitation room. A defibrillator should be readily available. The patient should be given 100% oxygen and the hyperkalaemia must be given urgent attention as this is immediately life threatening.

Consideration should be given to intubation and ventilation (avoiding suxamethonium!) for the following reasons:

1. He is agitated and therefore may not tolerate the necessary treatment (dialysis, i.v. infusions, central venous catheterisation and O_2 therapy)
2. He is hypoxaemic
3. He is hypoventilating because his PCO_2 is inappropriately high in the face of a metabolic acidosis

His haemodynamic state is complicated because he is hypotensive and bradycardic and has signs of left ventricular failure. The haemodynamic indices may be explained by the hyperkalaemia. Resolution of the hyperkalaemia may therefore produce a different haemodynamic picture. If the patient is still hypotensive the cause of his shock could be septic or cardiogenic in nature. A pulmonary artery catheter may resolve these issues.

7. *How would you treat a high K^+?*

Immediate measures to prevent cardiac arrest would be:

- 10–15 units of soluble insulin in 50 ml of 50% glucose i.v.
- 10 ml of 10% calcium chloride i.v. This stabilises the myocardium against arrhythmias

■ 50ml of 8.4% sodium bicarbonate will help correct acidosis and reduce the potassium level. However, the high sodium load should be considered and the minute ventilation needs to be adequate to excrete the CO_2 load produced otherwise intracellular acidosis may be worsened

■ Hyperventilation (if the patient is intubated) will also help reduce acidosis and therefore the hyperkalaemia

■ Nebulised β_2-agonists shift potassium into the cells

■ Avoidance of any potassium containing i.v. fluids e.g. Hartmanns

■ 15 g of calcium resonium qds p.o. (may take greater than 30 minutes to work). This acts as an ion exchange resin in the gut

These measures temporarily push the potassium back into the cells. This patient will need renal replacement therapy (ideally haemodialysis) to remove the excess potassium.

8. Which methods of renal replacement therapy do you know?

Haemodialysis
■ Efficient
■ Specialist centres only
■ A thin film of blood is passed by one side of a synthetic semi-permeable membrane whilst on the other side dialysate fluid is passed in the opposite direction. This creates a constant diffusion gradient for electrolytes.
■ The technique is performed intermittently for 4–6 hours
■ Anticoagulation is required

Haemofiltration
■ More cardiovascularly stable than haemodialysis
■ More widely available on intensive care units
■ Plasma water is removed by convection through a filter. The fluid is replaced with an appropriate electrolyte solution.
■ Less efficient than haemodialysis
■ Can be combined with dialysis (haemodiafiltration)
■ This technique is usually used continuously until the filter clots
■ Anticoagulation is required

Peritoneal dialysis
■ No need for sophisticated equipment
■ Principle is the same as haemodialysis but the membrane used is the peritoneal lining
■ 2 litres of sterile dialysate are placed into the peritoneal cavity via a catheter through the abdominal wall. In the acute situation this is drained out every hour. Electrolyte movement is by osmosis. Tonicity of the dialysate (and therefore degree of fluid removal) is determined by its glucose concentration

9. Why is he hypotensive?

This could be due to:

■ A cardiogenic cause, e.g. hyperkalaemia (causing bradycardia and myocardial dysfunction) or an alcoholic cardiomyopathy
■ Septic shock
■ Drug overdose

10. What about the treatment of rhabdomyolysis?

Treatment consists of management of the airway, breathing and circulation and correcting the underlying cause of the rhabdomyolysis. Further specific treatment of rhabdomyolysis is aimed at the prevention of renal failure.

The two factors that predispose to acute renal failure in the presence of myoglobinuria are **hypovolaemia** and **aciduria**. These two factors must therefore be addressed in the treatment:

■ Aim for urine output of 100 ml/hour
■ Dip urine hourly for pH and myoglobin testing
■ If urine pH < 7.0 give 100 mmol of sodium bicarbonate (can be repeated). Studies have shown bicarbonate therapy to be of benefit
■ If urine pH < 7.0 give acetazolamide 500 mg i.v. (can be repeated 4 hourly). This has not however been shown to be of consistent benefit
■ Mannitol can be used to promote a diuresis
■ Loop diuretics should be avoided as they acidify the urine
■ The depletion of extracellular iron by desferrioxamine may be of benefit
■ Allopurinol (xanthine oxidase inhibitor) has been used to try to decrease the hyperuricaemia associated with increased muscle protein breakdown

---

Mechanisms that underlie heme protein toxicity to the nephron

■ **Renal vasoconstriction.** Severe muscle damage results in gross ECF volume contraction. There is strong evidence that early volume repletion decreases the incidence of renal failure
■ **Intraluminal cast formation.** Myoglobin combines with tubular proteins to form casts. Acid pH of the tubular fluid favours the formation of these complexes. Alkaline conditions help to stop myoglobin-induced lipid peroxidation by stabilizing the reactive ferryl myoglobin complex that is responsible for causing oxidative damage. If the urinary pH is below 6.0, ferrihaemate (nephrotoxic) dissociates from myoglobin
■ **Heme-protein induced cytotoxicity.** Haemoglobin and myoglobin are usually reabsorbed into the proximal tubular cells by endocytosis. Inside the cell, porphyrin is metabolised producing free iron, which is converted into ferritin. When this pathway is overwhelmed the free iron builds up to levels that cause oxidant stress and cell damage

---

11. Is there a need for surgery in these patients?

Yes. Compartment syndrome must be looked for and treated. If Compartment syndrome is suspected then the compartmental pressures should be measured.

A normal pressure is less than 15 mmHg. A pressure of greater than 25 mmHg should trigger a surgical referral.

If Compartment syndrome is diagnosed, urgent fasciotomies are indicated. Debridement of any necrotic tissue is also frequently required.

Symptoms and signs of Compartment syndrome

- Pain – especially with passive flexion
- A swollen, hard limb
- Poor capillary refill
- Pulses may be present

References

Guidelines for the treatment of rhabdomyolysis. *Withington Hospital ICU*, 1999

Visweswaran P, Guntupalli J. Rhabdomyolysis. *Critical Care Clinics*, April 1999, Volume 15(2), p415–428

Long Case 15

'The elderly woman with kyphoscoliosis for an urgent cholecystectomy'

An 82-year-old lady is admitted to hospital with vomiting and jaundice. This is her second episode. She is known to have gallstones and the surgical team want to perform an open cholecystectomy.

She lives in a nursing home and has restricted mobility due to osteoarthritis. She is an ex-smoker and enjoys embroidery and knitting. Previous medical history includes postherpetic neuralgia and mild Alzheimer's disease.

Medications		
	Ibuprofen	400 mg t.d.s.
	Bendrofluazide	5 mg o.d.
	Carbamazepine	200 mg b.d.

O/E	
	Mildly confused, frail, jaundiced, kyphoscoliosis, temperature 37.7°C
	Weight 75 kg
	Pulse 100 irregular — Resp rate 16 bpm
	BP 160/84 mmHg — Generally quiet breath sounds
	HS normal — No wheeze audible
	Abdomen: tender with guarding in the right upper quadrant

Investigations			
	Hb 9.6 g/dl	Na 133 mmol/L	ALT 28 U/L (5–40)
	WCC 14.3 × 10⁹/L	K 3.3 mmol/L	AST 16 U/L (10–40)
	Plt 187 × 10⁹/L	U 11.6 mmol/L	Alk phos 238 U/L (25–115)
	MCV 84 fl	Cr 125 μmol/L	GGT 475 U/L (7–32)
		Glucose 6.4 mmol/L	Bilirubin 36 mmol/L (<17)

PFTs		
	FEV$_1$	1.8 L (2.3–3.6)
	FVC	2.2 L (3.9–5.0)
	FEV$_1$/ FVC ratio	82%
	TLC	4.6 L (5.6–7.5)
	DL$_{CO}$	7.8 mmol/kPa/min (8.2)

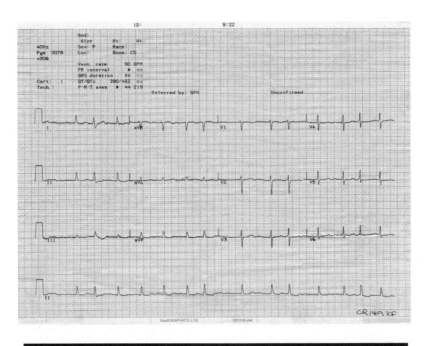

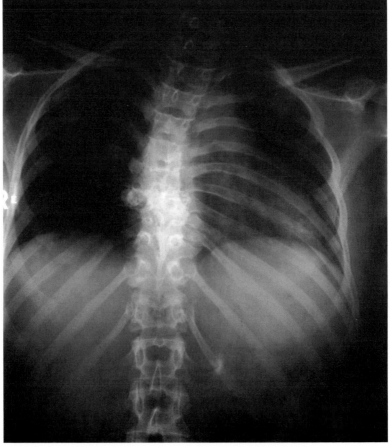

Questions

1. What do you think are the important features of this case?

This is an elderly lady with complex medical problems presenting for emergency upper abdominal surgery. The main issues of concern from the anaesthetic viewpoint are her atrial fibrillation, restrictive lung disease, fluid balance and postoperative analgesia.

2. What does the ECG show?

There is atrial fibrillation with a ventricular response of 90 beats per minute. The corrected QT interval is also slightly prolonged at 460 milliseconds, the normal being 420 milliseconds.

QT interval

- Measured from onset of QRS to end of T wave
- Can be difficult to measure precisely
- Normal QT_c (corrected for heart rate) < 420 milliseconds

Significance

- Predisposes to torsade de pointes ventricular tachycardia

Some causes of prolonged QT_c

- Congenital   Syndromes – Romano Ward, Jervell–Lange–Nielsen
- Acquired   Hypokalaemia, hypomagnesaemia, hypocalcaemia
                  Drugs, e.g. terfenadine, cisapride, erythromycin, amiodarone, amitryptiline, quinidine
                  Severe bradycardia
                  Acute MI

Treatment

- Magnesium
- Overdrive pacing

---

3. What does the CXR show?

There is significant kyphoscoliosis in keeping with the examination finding. A lateral chest X-ray would confirm this.

4. Would you like to comment on the pulmonary function tests?

All lung volumes are reduced but the FEV_1/FVC ratio is raised. This suggests a restrictive defect. The diffusion capacity for carbon monoxide is normal so it is unlikely to be pulmonary fibrosis. These results are compatible with the severe kyphoscoliosis seen clinically and on the chest X-ray.

See Appendix 1 for interpretation of commonly occurring PFTs.

---

5. What do you think about the haemoglobin?

The haemoglobin is low but the MCV is normal. If this was iron-deficiency anaemia secondary to Ibuprofen one would expect the MCV to be low as well. It may be anaemia of chronic disease.

6. Would you transfuse the patient pre-operatively?

The haemoglobin is 9.6 g/dL. She does not have clinically overt ischaemic heart disease and is unlikely to have significant blood loss intraoperatively. There is no current evidence to show that preoperative transfusion in patients with this level of anaemia has any effect on mortality. Blood transfusion is not without complications so, on balance, it would be reasonable to withhold transfusion. However, the surgeon should take extra care to avoid any unnecessary blood loss and blood should be available.

See Long Case 9 and short case on Massive Blood Transfusion.

7. Comment on the urea, electrolytes and liver function tests.

There is mild hyponatraemia and hypokalaemia, possibly secondary to bendrofluazide. The raised urea and creatinine suggest an element of dehydration as the urea is out of proportion to the creatinine. Although Hepato-renal syndrome is another possibility the level of jaundice makes it unlikely to be the cause.

The liver function tests show a raised bilirubin, alkaline phosphatase and GGT in keeping with obstructive jaundice. This is most likely to be secondary to gallstones although carbamazepine is also a recognised cause of an obstructive picture.

Causes of hypokalaemia

The list is enormous! Some of the more common causes to remember include:

- Diuretics
- Hyperaldosteronism   Liver failure
                        Heart failure
                        Nephrotic syndrome
- GI losses

8. Are there any other investigations you might want?

Coagulation profile: this lady has poor respiratory function and the nature of the surgery will result in significant postoperative pain and difficulty with deep breathing and coughing. She would therefore benefit from a regional block for postoperative analgesia but the liver function tests are abnormal.

9. What anaesthetic technique would you use for this lady?

Although this operation could, in theory, be performed under purely regional anaesthesia, the height of the epidural block necessary to undertake the operation with the patient awake is likely to result in respiratory embarrassment.

General anaesthesia with some form of regional block would be an appropriate technique. She would require a rapid sequence induction and intubation.

The options for postoperative analgesia include:

- Systemic opioids and NSAIDs (care with renal impairment)
- Thoracic epidural sited prior to induction but likely to be difficult in view of the kyphoscoliosis. She is also septic. One would weigh up the pros and cons
- Paravertebral block
- Intercostal blocks (risk of pneumothorax)
- Interpleural catheter

> Preferably choose a regional technique that you have performed before and can describe in detail.

Postoperative care on a high dependency unit with careful attention to oxygenation, fluid balance and analgesia is important.

Appendix 1

A system for interpreting and presenting chest X-rays

When faced with a chest X-ray in the heat of the examination it is vital to have a system of interpretation and presentation, particularly if the diagnosis does not jump out at you.

It is always difficult to know whether to present an X-ray starting with the diagnosis and following up with the supporting findings, or whether to use your system to present the findings and *then* reach a diagnosis.

For example: 'This chest X-ray shows the features of mitral stenosis which are ...' *or* 'There is a double heart border and calcification. ... These features suggest a diagnosis of mitral stenosis.'

In the long case you will have had a chance to view the chest X-ray and can therefore be more confident mentioning a diagnosis first. If the abnormality or diagnosis is 'barn-door' (e.g. large, cavitating lesion) then the examiners may not be impressed if you take 5 minutes to mention it! In the short cases you may be given chest X-rays that are more of a 'spot diagnosis' (such as pneumothorax) and you should try to mention the gross abnormality first. You should then use your system to make sure you do not miss other abnormalities (such as a bilateral pneumothorax!). Other chest X-rays may be more subtle (such as features of cardiac failure) and these may be better dealt with by using the systematic approach.

A suggested framework

Name/Sex	Look for breast shadows
Date	
PA/AP, lateral film	Clues: written on the film, 'mobile', scapulae, intubated, monitoring
Orientation i.e. left/right	
Rotation	Look at the heads of the clavicles
Penetration	Can you see the thoracic spine through the heart?
ET tube/tracheostomy	Comment on presence and position
Lines etc.	Comment on presence and position CVP – tip should be above the level of the carina. This ensures that it is outside the pericardium. PA catheter – the tip should be in the mid-zone. N/G, chest drains, ECG leads
Heart and mediastinum	Position, C/T ratio (not with AP), borders

Lungs	Expansion, hila–right higher than left normally
Bones and soft tissues	Fractures, metastases, surgical emphysema, etc.
'Areas easily missed'	Apices, behind the heart, below the diaphragm,the hila

An answer may begin:

'This is a chest X-ray of a female patient taken on **/**/**. It is an AP film as the patient is intubated. The film is not rotated and the penetration is adequate. The tip of the endotracheal tube is correctly placed. There is a central venous line in the right internal jugular vein and the tip lies in an appropriate position above the level of the carina. I cannot comment accurately on the heart size because of the projection of the film. There is no mediastinal shift. However, there is a small apical pneumothorax on the right, possibly as a consequence of insertion of the CVP line. The lung fields are otherwise clear.'

This approach is clearly not appropriate if you are presented with an obvious tension pneumothorax. In that situation it may be better to say:

'This is a left tension pneumothorax. There is a large left-sided pneumothorax with gross mediastinal shift. . .'

In summary, it may be best to tailor the technique of presentation to the type of abnormality seen and how confident you are about it.

Appendix 2

Interpretation of commonly occurring PFTs

Obstructive picture	$\downarrow$ FEV$_1$
	$\downarrow$ FVC
	$\downarrow$ FEV$_1$/FVC ratio (normal around 75%)
	$\downarrow$ FEF$_{25-75}$ (forced expiratory flow)
	$\downarrow/\rightarrow$DL$_{CO}$
	(FEF$_{25-75}$ is representative of small airways)
Restrictive picture	$\downarrow$ FEV$_1$
	$\downarrow$ FVC
	$\uparrow$ FEV$_1$/FVC ratio
	$\downarrow/\rightarrow$DL$_{CO}$

Interpretation of DL$_{CO}$ and K$_{CO}$

- Carbon monoxide transfer factor (DL$_{CO}$) is reduced in conditions that damage the alveolar capillary membrane, e.g. pulmonary fibrosis and in conditions where lung surface area is reduced, e.g. emphysema and pneumonectomy. It is also reduced in anaemia and ventilation/perfusion mismatch
- K$_{CO}$ (= DL$_{CO}$ corrected for lung volume) remains low in pulmonary fibrosis but is higher in emphysema and pneumonectomy where it is the total lung surface area that is reduced

Flow-volume loops in large airway obstruction

Variable extrathoracic obstruction, e.g. goitre
- Inspiratory limb flattened (normally semicircular) as trachea collapses on inspiration
- Expiration OK as trachea 'pushed' open

Variable intrathoracic obstruction
- Expiratory limb flattened as trachea 'pushed' closed
- Inspiratory limb OK as trachea 'pulled' open

Fixed large airway obstruction
- Both inspiratory and expiratory limbs are flattened

Index

Abbreviations used in subheadings in the index are: AAA = abdominal aortic aneurysm; AF = atrial fibrillation; COPD = chronic obstructive pulmonary disease; CSF = cerebrospinal fluid; DVT = deep vein thrombosis; ICP = intracranial pressure; ICU = intensive care unit; RBBB = right bundle branch block; RTA = road traffic accident; SIRS = Systemic Inflammatory Response Syndrome; TURP = transurethral resection of the prostate; WPW Syndrome = Wolff–Parkinson–White syndrome